AVA
D I

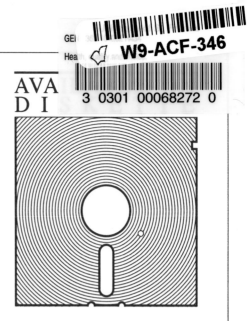

EASY REFERENCE
AND COMPARISON FOR ANALYSIS
ON PERSONAL COMPUTERS

The 120 000 figures provided in this publication and many other data are available on diskette.

If you are a frequent user of the data, analyst or decision-maker, you need

OECD HEALTH DATA / ÉCO-SANTÉ OCDE

price: **FF 2 250   £ 250   US$ 400   DM 680**

(special rates for academic circles, government bodies, hospital boards)

The user-friendly software on the diskette not only gives immediate access to more than 200 000 statistics but also permits the easy construction of tables, charts and graphs in line with your own requirements. Data can be exported for use in other software programmes. OECD area and European maps can be accessed instantaneously.

A network version is also available.

Send your order or request for a free information brochure to:

OECD in Paris (Electronic Editions),
its Publications and Information Centres
or the distributor in your country.

ORDER FORM

❏ I wish to order

OECD HEALTH DATA / ÉCO-SANTÉ OCDE

at the price of:

FF 2 250   £ 250   US$ 400   DM 680

❏ Send invoice: official order attached   ❏ Payment is enclosed

Name _____

Address _____

_____

Country _____

Signature _____ Date _____

HEALTH POLICY STUDIES No. 4

HEALTH:
QUALITY
AND CHOICE

ORGANISATION FOR ECONOMIC CO-OPERATION AND DEVELOPMENT

ORGANISATION FOR ECONOMIC CO-OPERATION AND DEVELOPMENT

Pursuant to Article 1 of the Convention signed in Paris on 14th December 1960, and which came into force on 30th September 1961, the Organisation for Economic Co-operation and Development (OECD) shall promote policies designed:

— to achieve the highest sustainable economic growth and employment and a rising standard of living in Member countries, while maintaining financial stability, and thus to contribute to the development of the world economy;

— to contribute to sound economic expansion in Member as well as non-member countries in the process of economic development; and

— to contribute to the expansion of world trade on a multilateral, non-discriminatory basis in accordance with international obligations.

The original Member countries of the OECD are Austria, Belgium, Canada, Denmark, France, Germany, Greece, Iceland, Ireland, Italy, Luxembourg, the Netherlands, Norway, Portugal, Spain, Sweden, Switzerland, Turkey, the United Kingdom and the United States. The following countries became Members subsequently through accession at the dates indicated hereafter: Japan (28th April 1964), Finland (28th January 1969), Australia (7th June 1971), New Zealand (29th May 1973) and Mexico (18th May 1994). The Commission of the European Communities takes part in the work of the OECD (Article 13 of the OECD Convention).

Publié en français sous le titre :
LA SANTÉ : QUALITÉ ET CHOIX

FOREWORD

The art of public policy-making lies essentially in careful evaluation of the various trade-offs and their implications. Many, and often highly conflicting, interests have to be considered. Policy then tends to be an informed compromise between the prevailing pressures. Ironically, perhaps, in their zeal to defend their values, the various protagonists may not realise that their distinct and particular goals can often be achieved simultaneously. The formulation of health care policy is a prime example of this process.

At the heart of current debate is the question "Quality at what cost?" On the one hand are the patients, whose chief interest is in a desirable outcome: a cure, a remission, the attainment of good health. Equally concerned that their intervention improves the well-being of their patients are the medical and paramedical practitioners. Planners too are keen to improve the effectiveness of the systems which link the input with the output. These various agents have much the same goals. On the other hand, there are inevitable financial constraints.

This volume, the fourth in a series devoted to comparative analysis of health care systems, addresses several facets of the quality issue – all too often seen as clashing with principles of economic efficiency. Is quality possible where financial considerations weigh heavily on all systems? The six authors in the volume come from a variety of backgrounds and bring to the question the multiplicity of their experiences. In many ways they concur: it is plainly evident that medical progress, like medical facilities themselves, requires considerable resources. But the choice of appropriate technologies, well thought out targeting, new ways and means of allocating both human and financial resources might actually contribute to expenditure restraint. As our experience widens, it may emerge that those who insisted that "quality costs" were only half correct. In some cases, quality costs less.

Earlier drafts of the essays benefited from comments from the OECD Working Party on Social Policy. Like the investigations reported on in *Health Care Systems in Transition* (OECD, Paris, 1990) they are part of a broadly-based investigation into the determinants of health care spending in Member countries and the strategies pursued to enhance the "value for money" precept now emerging as the guiding principle of contemporary health policies. Financial support for these essays was provided by the United States Health Care Financing Administration.

This report is published on the authority of the Secretary General of the OECD.

T.J. Alexander
Director for Education,
Employment, Labour and
Social Affairs

3

About the authors

Anne-Marie WORNING, now at the Regional Office for Europe of the World Health Organisation, Copenhagen, Denmark, was an independent consultant at the time of preparing this essay.

Miriam WILEY is director of the Health Policy Research Centre in the Economic and Social Research Institute, Dublin, and a consultant for the European Community and the World Health Organisation.

Harold LUFT is a professor of health economics at the Institute for Health Policy Studies, School of Medicine, University of San Francisco.

Markus SCHNEIDER, director of BASYS, in Augsburg, Germany, is a consultant for the European Community.

Michael DICKSON is dean of the College of Pharmacy, South Carolina University, United States.

Helena BRUS, an industry economist, was an independent consultant working at the time of preparing this essay.

TABLE OF CONTENTS

INTRODUCTION

During the century following the intervention of governments in setting up a variety of health insurance approaches, beginning in Prussia, spreading rapidly to other European countries and continents, the health systems of the OECD countries have experienced distinct phases of development. In the beginning, medical services played only a modest role. With the advent of antibiotics and other therapeutic advances, medical consumption became more important than the income maintenance side of health insurance.

Since World War II three concerns have become dominant:
- the search for a universal coverage against the financial consequences of disease,
- the search for control over expenditure,
- the search for quality and for a different empowerment structure.

If medical coverage was not as yet universal in the OECD area when the oil shock broke out, the access problem had, however, largely been solved. Hence, there was a shift towards efficiency and towards a slowing down in the growth of the preceding era's rapidly escalating expenditures. Since signs were showing of the ability to bring expenditure closer in line with affordability constraints, attention began to focus, in the latter half of the 1980s, on greater effectiveness: medical procedures are expected to yield a positive outcome. Simply providing suppliers with the financial resources required no longer suffices. A contractual relationship between "purchasers", acting on behalf of consumers, and producers has emerged as a tool to reconcile productivity and achievement.

Lack of quality can turn out to be costly. It generates unnecessary patient suffering, it wastes resources. Effectiveness remains, however, a difficult operational concept. Even now, good health is only measured by its absence. Society moves by a trial and error process. All countries appear committed, however, to reconciling four objectives: equity (defined as the easy access of all to required health services regardless of income), efficiency (a better allocation of resources within limits of affordability), effectiveness (the allocation of resources for improvements in the health status), empowerment (the patient participates in decisions relating to the improvement of his/her health).

The implementation of the health reforms is a bumpy road: vested powers are perturbed by the new approaches to delivering and financing health care. Society still has difficulties in assessing objectives. For changes to make an impression, time is needed. Pressures for change have increased and reforms have started almost everywhere.

OECD's input in the debate relates to the dual objectives of monitoring changes across subject areas and country trends. In this publication, non-quality is perceived as a cost: hospital acquired infection, for instance, induced disability spells and generates sizeable outlays; it can often be prevented at low cost. For a contractual relationship between purchaser and provider to exist hospital outputs need to be carefully defined. Services provided are only efficient if the purchaser and often the user know what they can expect. Services provided by hospitals are more diverse than in industrialised establishments of equivalent size. Indicators such as numbers of days or numbers of beds do not give information on the diversity of services provided. Reforms have started; the description below does not catch up with their speed but is a useful assessment.

Another essay points out the utility of knowing what the consumption of pharmaceutical products comprises. Do inter-country differences depend on the total amount spent on health care? Where it is identified, is overconsumption not general for all therapeutic categories? By raising the question in numeral terms, an essay in this volume contributes to a rigorous comparative dimension of the issue. The similarity in behaviour, in spite of some surprising disparities, is not only observed in terms of quantities apparently consumed, but it is also found in price trends. Differences have not been eradicated by market internationalisation. Consumption and price trends somehow need to be rationalised.

New forms of health delivery and financing have to be imagined in hospitals and elsewhere. What applies at sub-systemic level is found necessary at systems level; Germany has felt the need to make regular amendments to its system. Society is in constant evolution: why should this not be so for health care systems too? Forty years later, have the structures been adapted to efficacy and efficiency requirements inconceivable at the end of the Second World War?

This publication comprises exploratory work on health care systems undertaken by the OECD over the last few years. Some of it refer to a group of Member states, others to narrower geographic boundaries. In political debates there is often a contradiction between quality and economy. The following analyses show that the prevention of complications, the development of alternative paths to care, greater transparency, can lead to a more appropriate level of medical consumption and to the joint pursuit of quality of service and user satisfaction.

These essays are a small stepping stone in the conceptualisation of health care systems. Supply and demand constraints require priorities. These issues generally approached at national level may also be viewed in a broader perspective. Each author had to be imaginative in his own setting. An international perspective permits to share common problems and common practices.

STRATEGIES FOR REDUCTION OF HOSPITAL-ACQUIRED INFECTIONS
A model for quality development

by

Anne Marie Worning

The following is an overview of the medical, social and economic consequences of hospital-acquired infections (HAI) – or nosocomial infections (NI). The focus on strategies for HAI prevention, leads to offer a model for quality improvement generally. While the aim is to alert health economists and policy-makers to a specific problem, it is also to motivate them to allocate the resources necessary to establish preventive programmes at the local, regional or national level.

A few words about quality in health care

The last five years have seen a renewed focus on the notion of quality in health care. A whole vocabulary has re-emerged to surround us: "Quality assurance", "quality assessment", "quality development", "continuous quality improvement", "total quality management" and the like. The terminology and its basic underlying concepts stem from the industrial sector and date to the early 1960s. Yet despite this, the comprehensive model of quality assurance (QA) in health care has only recently begun to interest large portions of the medical profession.[1] This model, with it three-part focus on structure, process and outcome, is still the corner-stone of QA in health care.[2]

What is the aim of quality assurance?

When clients enter a health care system, a cascade of processes is instigated aiming to produce a specific outcome – namely to give these clients some benefit or assistance.

In the current health care debate where *quality* is used as an *ad hoc* term by all, it becomes important to remember that the overall goal of health care is neither to build or to remodel a system, nor to quantify, analyse or audit the process – unless these activities can be shown to have some beneficial effect on the outcome for the patient. If the overall goal of health care is to improve health, it would then be logical to measure the success of activities in terms of outcome measures or outcome indicators.

Trends in quality assurance: the outcome approach

General outcomes include mortality, morbidity and indices such as "quality adjusted life years" (QALY), and scores for new-borns (APGAR), etc. Some of these measures, although related to outcome, may be meaningless for the individual; because of their multi-factorial origin, they are, in many cases, too insensitive to point towards specific quality problems. On the other hand, to determine differences in these outcomes over a time span, the volume of data to be collected needs to be quite large. This often makes the time-frame too long for the remedial actions to benefit the individual. However, continuous monitoring of such outcomes are important for detecting the large areas of the health care system which need revising. For example, infant mortality remains largely unchanged over time in Eastern Europe, the rate being triple that of Western Europe.[3] Such information is therefore valuable for future health strategy and policy decisions.

One may also choose to look at a tracer condition, and define criteria and standards of good care for that specific condition. This method does not focus on individuals, but screens a population for the tracer and in this way detects undiagnosed cases, measures the gap between delivered and professed care and assesses the number of preventable and poor outcomes. This method has been used for tracing anaemia and diabetes, for example.[4] The merit of the method is its focus on the entire health care system. Tracer conditions studied should have a relatively high prevalence in the population as well as having important health care consequences. They should be well defined (both with regard to diagnosis and treatment) and not heavily influenced by non-medical factors.

Due to the magnitude and cost of conducting tracer programmes, outcomes of single events are often preferred for study. These so-called sentinel events normally focus on things that go wrong. Sentinel events can refer to single unique events (such as maternal death[5] or death in the operating room) but they can also be symptoms of a wider set of problems, such as hospital acquired infections (HAI).

Until recently the tendency has been to focus on evaluation of the structure and process of health care. The last five years, however, have seen a clear shift towards developing valid methods for measuring outcomes.[6, 7] In this swing of the pendulum, some suggest that if the outcome is good, then the process by which it was reached is not important. This is an over-simplification: a poor process, despite good outcomes, may waste resources and expose patients to unnecessary risks. Furthermore, by improving the process, even better outcomes might be achieved.

The structure, process and outcome are therefore intertwined and should be looked at in this light. The outcome, whether exceptionally good or poor, is always the result of some processes carried out in a specific setting or structure. Poor outcomes might therefore be used as "pointers for investigation". One can choose to study that part of the process or elements of the structure which seem the most likely cause of a poor result, and then institute remedial actions. Conversely, one can identify institutions or individuals that have excellent outcomes and try to adopt elements of their process and structure.

What is a HAI?

In general terms, a hospital-acquired infection (HAI) is just that an infection is acquired by a person in contact with a hospital. In medical terms, a HAI is defined as an infection which the patient neither had nor was incubating at the time of admission to hospital.

A major health care problem

HAIs constitute a major health care problem in both developed and developing countries. In both epidemic and endemic form, they are among the leading causes of morbidity and mortality in hospitalised patients. HAIs prolong hospitalisation, add appreciably to the cost of the original illness, and take their toll in human lives, illness and disability. It is no exaggeration to say that between 5 and 10% of all patients entering hospital in the developed world acquire one or more nosocomial infections (NIs).[8] In addition, NIs present not only a risk to patients, but also to hospital staff and visitors who are in constant contact with infectious micro-organisms present in the hospital environment.

Major improvements to prevent HAIs have occurred over the past 50 years such as the widespread use of disinfectants and the development of potent antibiotics. These have significantly reduced the frequency of epidemics due to streptococcal and staphylococcal bacteria. However, the level of HAIs is still high – and can be expected to remain so – unless effective strategies for HAI prevention and control are introduced.

This being noted, it is self-evident that HAIs pose serious implications for the patient, the health care professionals, and health care systems:

- For the patient, a HAI is an infection which was unexpected, a risk of which he or she was unaware, and with consequences about which he or she was probably not informed. A patient admitted to surgery would be at rights to demand immediate cure, expecting no residual or added disability, and would want to return quickly to normal life. The possibility of such a patient returning to stable social and working conditions may be shattered if admission to hospital is complicated by a severe HAI.

- For the medical profession, a HAI will mean further diagnostic and therapeutic strategies and possibly additional interventions and increased demand for service.
- For the hospital management, a HAI will increase costs in the form of additional bed days, extra use of resources and changes in planning.
- For the family, a HAI may imply delayed homecoming of a relative. It may also imply that the afflicted person may be subject to a permanent handicap.
- For society at large, HAIs may mean a loss of lives and/or an increased – indeed lifelong – demand for social welfare in the form of extra pension, etc.

An example

The widespread implications of HAI at different levels may be best illustrated by the following example: an elderly patient is admitted to hospital with the expectation of being cured of a severe hip pain. The medical profession expects a safe and efficacious hip joint replacement of high technical quality, using the latest available technology (*e.g.* new joint made from a combination of metal and ceramic material). The hospital management expects total recovery and a speedy discharge from hospital, followed by ambulatory physiotherapy. The family expects the person to return home with the opportunity to enjoy life with increased physical, psychological and social well-being. Society expects the patient to become self-reliant once again with no requirement for extra services and expects him/her to continue as an active member of society. Fortunately, these anticipations most often culminate in reality.

In contrast, however, the patient may spend as many as two extra weeks in hospital in mild cases of infection in the surgical wound. In more severe cases of wound infection, there may be a need to reoperate with removal of the entire hip joint or parts of the prosthesis. The patient may acquire a blood stream infection which, despite intensive antibiotic therapy, may prove fatal. If the patient survives a severe infection, he or she may return to the family and local community with an even greater handicap than before. He or she may even be permanently confined to a wheelchair. If a completely stiff limb or amputation is the end result of such an infection, rehousing and vast changes in social support will likely be necessary. In HAI cases the hospital management must cope with extended hospitalisation: up to a tenfold increase in expected hospital costs and severe demands on medical services. The patient once handicapped, but productive, may become a client with an increased need for health care services, or even a candidate for lifelong social welfare. The overall loss to society is enormous in both economic and psychosocial terms.

Furthermore, when addressing the HAI problem, the changing demography must be considered. Hospital-based treatment of the increasing number of elderly by means of advanced technology will have its impact, in terms of accelerated HAI problems.

HAIs: A budget drain

The demand for hospital services today around the world is increasing. For most countries this is not simultaneously complemented by an overall increase in the health care budget. In such settings, it therefore becomes important to ensure that the money spent on health care results in the highest possible level of quality. The economic drain on the health care sector created by HAIs is enormous It can, however, be reduced, as there are established programmes for reduction of HAIs, the impact of which is well documented. Introduction of effective means to reduce HAIs would provide a valuable way of releasing economic resources to other areas of the health care system. Efforts in the field of prevention of HAIs are therefore not to be considered in isolation but should be seen as one of many activities with a far-reaching impact on the entire health care delivery system.

What can we do to control HAIs?

Since HAI control or prevention is an area where methodologies have been developed, tested and documented, there is reason for optimism. Much can be done to reduce the risk of HAI despite the fact that not all HAIs are preventable. Some speak of the "irreducible minimum".

During the last decade it has become evident that up to one-third of all HAIs are avoidable by adhering to stringent hygienic routines and by implementing effective surveillance programmes and preventive strategies.[9]

Once low levels of infection have been reached, one may choose to monitor these routinely to ensure that the standard is kept up in recognition of the fact that once low levels are reached, further improvement may prove not to be cost-effective. For example, a reduction in wound infection rate following hernia surgery from 2 to 1% may require such enormous resources that the benefit is considered minimal in relation to the effort and cost required. Critical choices in this area will therefore have to be made and the best value for money sought. However, it is to date unclear who should make these choices, *e.g.* physicians, patients, or governments, and with whom the responsibility actually lies?

How are HAIs measured?

In order to verify that preventive strategies are functioning, the rate of HAIs has to be measured accurately. Two different types of surveys are usually carried out to estimate the occurrence of HAIs, *i.e.* prevalence surveys and incidence surveys, and the corresponding results are reported as prevalence and incidence rates. These measures are not the same and should therefore not be directly compared.[10]

In the case of *prevalence surveys,* hospitalised patients (or patient records) are examined at one point in time. A prevalence rate, therefore, reflects the situation as given in a hospital/ward/region/country at one specific point in time and hence gives a "snapshot" image of the situation.

Incidence surveys study the occurrence of new cases of HAIs during a defined period of time. These can be carried out retrospectively by using patient records after discharge or prospectively by following patients from the time of admission.

It should be noted that method of data collection, selection of study population, and duration of survey, have immense influence on the resulting incidence and prevalence rates.

Both incidence and prevalence surveys are normally carried out only during hospitalisation. However, some types of NIs only become clinically active after discharge despite the fact that they were acquired during hospitalisation. This is especially true for surgical wound infections (SWIs). With the current tendency to discharge patients earlier, *e.g.* 1-2 days post-operatively for minor surgery, the number of infections not taken into account can be quite large. Approximately 25-50% of all SWIs occur after discharge and these are therefore not accounted for in the majority of studies reported here.[11, 12] There is a fair risk that the proportion of unregistered SWIs may be increasing as the volume of surgery being performed as day surgery is growing. Reported low rates of SWI, relying solely on hospital-based surveillance, may therefore be giving a false sense of security: this is an area that warrants further in-depth investigation. Third-party payers and regulatory agencies in the OECD area at present monitoring the bulk of day surgery should emphasize the need for out-patient surveillance, in order to get a clear view of the level of post-operative complications connected to this type of surgical practice.

The scope of the problem

The lack of uniformity in reporting HAIs and the absence of accepted international standards make comparison difficult and sometimes meaningless. There is currently no basis for exact multicentre or multinational comparisons and only rough overall pointers to the size of the problem can be identified.

Therefore, with due caution paid to relating data from hospitals in one country to those in others (and making global extrapolations), it is estimated that out of the 190 million persons admitted to hospitals throughout the world each year, a minimum of 5% (more than 9 million persons) acquire a hospital infection. Among these 9 million patients, 1 million deaths occur directly or indirectly from NIs. This is a very conservative estimate made by the World Health Organisation in 1980.[13]

There is a wide range, from about 5 to 15%, in mean *prevalence* of HAIs in reported studies.[8] The inter-institutional range reported from multicentre or multinational studies has shown even greater variations. For example, the inter-institutional range for Thailand was 2-26% while for Norway it was 5-21%. Graph 1 includes nosocomial infection prevalence results from large national studies covering Australia, Belgium, Czech and Slovak Republics, Denmark, Italy, Norway and Thailand.[14-22] The mean

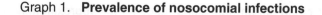

Graph 1. Prevalence of nosocomial infections

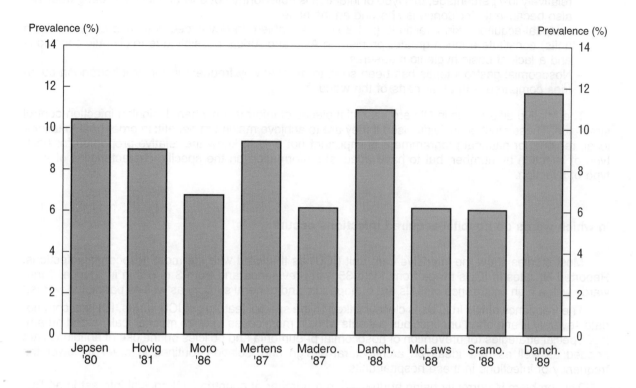

Prevalence (%)

Prevalence (%)

| Jepsen '80 | Hovig '81 | Moro '86 | Mertens '87 | Madero. '87 | Danch. '88 | McLaws '88 | Sramo. '88 | Danch. '89 |

prevalence rate is seen to be within the range of 6-11%. These studies represent some of the large national studies conducted during the last ten years. However, it is interesting to see that such global figures are still in line with more recent data from a very large study in Spain (EPINE 1990). This study is based on reporting from 123 hospitals and includes more than 38 000 patients. In this study the overall prevalence rate was found to be 9.87%.[23]

International studies demonstrate a wide range in values from 1 to 15% in the *incidence* of NIs. However, if small surveys featuring specific wards or those of a pilot nature are excluded, then the incidence of NIs lies around 4%.[8] In reality, this means that the mean risk of acquiring an infection during hospitalisation is roughly 4%. However, what the result is to the patient is very largely dependent on the type of infection.

The most common HAIs

The three most prevalent HAIs are urinary tract infections (UTI), respiratory tract infections (RTI) and surgical wound infections (SWI). Fewer in number but also important are blood stream infections, gastrointestinal infections and skin infections.

The relative proportion by number of different types of infection varies with the age of the population and geographical location.

- In Europe and North America, for example, where the hospital population is characterised as being elderly, urinary tract infections account for approximately 50% of all HAIs.[24]
- Globally, SWIs are the second most common NI and seem to be the most evenly distributed type of HAI both in terms of age and global occurrence. On a global basis, SWIs constitute approximately 25% of all HAIs.[25]
- Respiratory tract infections (of which pneumonia is the most severe) have increased in number during the past decade and constitute around 15-20% of all HAIs.

- Bacteraemias (or blood stream infections) account for approximately 5% of HAIs. Despite the relatively low percentage, this type of infection is noteworthy not only because it is dangerous but also because its incidence is showing an increase.
- Hospital-acquired skin infections (not a severe problem in developed countries except in burn units) constitute a much greater problem in Asia and Africa, possibly due to climatic conditions and a lack of basic hygienic measures.
- Nosocomial gastroenteritis has been seen to be relatively frequent in the Mediterranean countries compared with other parts of the world.[25]

The relative differences in NIs are essential pieces of information when designing infection-control strategies. These must be individualised if they are to achieve maximum benefit: in order best to tailor a local, regional or national programme it is important not only to know the relative proportion for each type of infection by number, but to have adequate information on the specific characteristics of each type of infection.

In which wards do hospital-acquired infections occur?

Most studies show the intensive care unit (ICU) as the ward with the most nosocomial infections. Reported NI rates in ICUs range from 11 to 35% in prevalence and from 3 to 5% in incidence. Other wards with a high occurrence of HAIs are orthopaedic and general surgery as well as paediatric wards.[8]

The frequency of NIs in ICUs is closely linked to the special features of ICU wards. ICUs accommodate severely ill and often unconscious patients who, in most cases, require mechanically-aided breathing. Special strategies for prevention of nosocomial pneumonia and policies on the use of antibiotics are needed as well as new ideas on architectural design and isolation routines in order to lower the frequency of infections in these hospital units.

This problem is currently being addressed in a number of countries. Of special interest is an EC-funded project (COMAC-EURO.NIs) which aims to give valid estimates on the rate of NIs in ICUs as well as to develop specific strategies for reducing nosocomial pneumonia in ICUs.[26]

Distribution of nosocomial infections by age

As illustrated in Graph 2, there is a higher frequency of HAIs in the very young and older population groups, and a more even distribution in the adult population. This is also reflected in the types of infections which occur. Pneumonia is prevalent in the very young and the very old, while urinary tract infections are mostly confined to the aged.

Characteristics of the different types of HAIs

a) **Urinary tract infections** are the most common NIs and therefore require special attention. Of these infections, 80% are linked to instrumentation of the urinary tract and in this respect the most common procedure is the placement of indwelling bladder catheters.[24] Many other factors, however, influence the development of nosocomial urinary tract infections, e.g. initial diagnosis, patient age, underlying diseases, surgical procedures, duration of surgery and recurrence of the infection. Nosocomial urinary tract infections are, in most cases, not severe, do not significantly prolong hospitalisation, and can usually be treated by means of antibiotics. This type of NI is seldom associated with acute or long-term complications or even with permanent disability.

The most important factor concerning this type of infection is its link to the placement of urinary catheters. The general use of bladder catheters is too widespread and strategies to reduce their use will have an immediate beneficial effect. The use of urinary catheters can never be totally abandoned, but studies which clearly define the target group and which evaluate alternative solutions are mandatory. The reduced use of urinary catheters will involve a behavioural change by both health care professionals and patients.

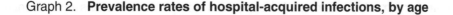

Graph 2. **Prevalence rates of hospital-acquired infections, by age**

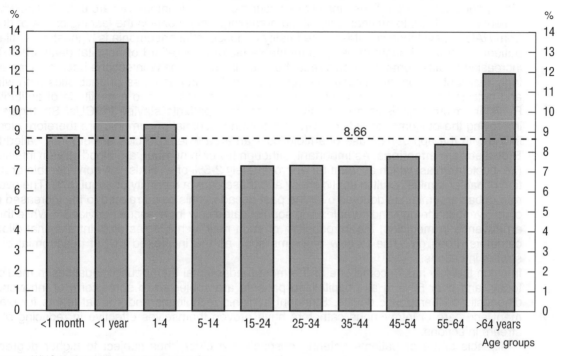

8.66

Age groups

<1 month <1 year 1-4 5-14 15-24 25-34 35-44 45-54 55-64 >64 years

Source: WHO Hospital Infection Prevalence Survey.

b) **Surgical wound infections (SWIs)** are the second most common HAI and although they account only for approximately 25% by number, they consume 60% of added bed days and 40% of the total added cost of HAIs.[27] In addition, SWIs are very important because of their association with high mortality and morbidity. Fortunately, in most cases of general surgery, the SWI is superficial, and only delays the healing process and scarring of the wound, accompanied by physical and psychological discomfort. In some cases it may be necessary to perform extra minor operations such as opening of the wound for drainage purposes both during the spell of hospitalisation and/or the period of ambulatory convalescence.

The dangerous type of SWIs is the deep infections. In these, the infection is spread to deeper tissue (*e.g.* muscles, joints and vessels), and these may carry as high a mortality rate as 10-20%. In some specialities, such as vascular surgery, SWIs are extremely serious. Graft infections are a paramount problem in 1-6% of patients undergoing peripheral revascularisation. Mortality rates as high as 75% have been reported in patients with infected prostheses of the aorta, and the survivors have a 75% incidence of limb loss.[28]

SWIs are also important in orthopaedic surgery, especially in cases of implantation of new joints – a fast developing surgical field. Severe wound infections following knee and hip prostheses carry a mortality risk of approximately 2-6%. The risk of permanent handicap in the form of joint stiffness and chronic pain is also very high in these types of operations. Of the patients contracting any kind of wound infection after knee operations, up to 50% may suffer some form of permanent disability.[29, 30]

Joint prostheses have become an indispensable part of the surgeon's armamentarium, and disabling chronic diseases such as arthritis have been revolutionised by metallic/plastic/ceramic whole joint replacement. Pins, screws and plates are also intimate parts of fracture treatment. The trend to use more "hardware" and the increased demand for orthopaedic and vascular surgery are expected to continue as the "greying" of the population increases. In this context, it is important to implement specific strategies for reducing SWIs as they have especially severe repercussions in these two surgical specialities.

c) **Respiratory tract infections.** Although respiratory tract infections only account for approximately 15-20% of all HAIs, lower respiratory tract infection in the form of nosocomial pneumonia is becoming an increasing problem and is especially prevalent in the very young and the older population groups. These infections occur most often in intensive care units (ICUs) where patients are subject to mechanically-aided breathing. Pneumonia is the leading cause of death from HAIs in developed countries. The fatality of nosocomial pneumonia is highest in ventilated patients, and it is thought to be an attributable factor in one-third of hospital deaths.[31, 32] The increasing fatality from pneumonia must be seen in light of these infections becoming increasingly resistant to normal antibiotic therapy. Due to the abundant use of antibiotics both within and outside hospital, micro-organisms emerge that are resistant to a multitude of antibiotics. Resistant micro-organisms are mainly cultured from patients staying in ICUs. Strategies for improving the outcome for patients who contract nosocomial pneumonia are therefore closely linked with the appropriate use of antibiotics – an area where policies are urgently called for.

d) **Blood stream infections.** As important, although fewer in number, are blood stream infections (*i.e.* bacteraemias) which account for approximately 2-5% of all HAIs.[33] A considerable proportion of bacteraemias result in septic shock and these carry a mortality of about 30%. The overall rate of bacteraemia has doubled over the past decade – this being related to the increased use of intravenous therapy and complex and sophisticated new intravascular devices.[34] While this is an advance in medicine, the introduction of such new technologies (*e.g.* intraluminal dilation catheters) does give rise to new problems such as the increased risk of nosocomial blood stream infections.

Infusion therapy has become one of the most fundamental therapeutic modalities in medicine today, and over 50% of all hospitalised patients are subjected to some form of intravenous diagnostic or therapeutic device. Stringent hygienic techniques and special teams for placement and care of intravenous catheters have proven themselves effective in reducing blood stream infections.

A sizeable share or patients entering hospitals are older, thus subject to higher degree of comorbidities and poorer health status. This is in part due to the ability of the ambulatory system better to deal with the lighter cases. As a result, the problem of hospital-acquired infections related to the use of intravascular devices will probably continue to rise. Much research is needed to study the more varied use of intravascular devices in order better to define which patient group, method, length of time, and what specific device is the most appropriate.

Appropriate use of antibiotics in hospitals

Prevention of HAIs is closely connected to the appropriate use of antibiotics. One important component of infection control is the prophylactic use of antibiotics during surgery. However, it must be remembered that this is only one aspect of antibiotic utilisation. There is no doubt today that the use of antibiotics as surgical prophylaxis is beneficial in preventing SWIs, especially in connection with surgical procedures carrying a high risk of contamination, such as colorectal surgery.

It is only over the past decade, however, that the appropriate and rational use of antibiotic prophylaxis in surgery has been delineated. Following the publication of clinical trials during the 1950s and 1960s (which showed no increased benefit of antibiotic prophylaxis) some confusion existed concerning the efficacy of this practice. However, errors were found in the study design of these early efforts (non-randomisation, lack of control, inappropriate timing of initial antibiotic administration, incorrect choice of antimicrobial agents) and most of these problems have been clarified.

The most significant problem was timing of antibiotic prophylaxis. The classical work of Burke, which demonstrated the crucial relationship between timing of antibiotic administration and prophylactic efficacy ought to have had an immediate impact on changing practice.[35] However, this was not the case and so-called "prophylactic" antibiotics are still being given after completion of the operation. This is not only an ineffective procedure, but also a waste of resources.

The principles of antibiotic prophylaxis are, in general, related to administering

- the correct drug;
- to the correct type of patient;
- at the correct time;

– for the correct duration;
– using the correct route of administration.[36]

Although guidelines for the correct use of prophylaxis exist, audits of actual practice often display an appreciable gap between intended and actual practice. This has recently been illustrated in a large survey carried out in Belgium where the preliminary results show that approximately half of the patients receiving prophylactic antibiotic treatments have these administered for more than 24 hours,[37] contrary to accepted standards of practice and explicit guidelines.

In relation to local microflora, the widespread use of antibiotics has resulted in the emergence of multi-resistant strains and increasingly more potent and expensive antibiotics are having to be used.[38]

The use of antibiotics varies considerably from country to country. For example, in some countries aminoglycosides, a family of potent but potentially dangerous group of antibiotics, are restricted to hospital use; in other countries these antibiotics are freely used in primary health care settings.[39] While the prevalence of multi-resistant bacterial strains isolated from hospitals in countries with restricted use of potent antibiotics is normally low, countries with very liberal use of antibiotics outside the hospital have a higher risk of serious epidemics due to an abundance of multi-resistant bacterial strains. Such data make a strong case for including information on antibiotic consumption in relevant surveillance data in order better to direct antibiotic policy at the regional and national levels.

Antibiotic policies at the national level which include restricted lists (selected drugs for use in primary health care and hospitals) and continuous surveillance of changes in prevalent micro-organisms and their resistance patterns, are necessary for appropriate antibiotic utilisation.

There is little doubt that there is a general over-utilisation of antibiotics in hospital and primary health care settings. It has been estimated that up to 50% of the total use of antibiotics in hospitals is either unnecessary, inappropriately administered or given in the wrong dose. Therefore, implementation of effective antibiotic policies could be a very important means to improve the quality of care as well as saving money. Corner stones of such policies would include:
– abandonment of unnecessary prescription of new and expensive antibiotics;
– abandonment of unnecessary prophylaxis;
– development of restricted antibiotic lists; and
– annual analyses of local antibiotic use in relation to changes in local microflora.[40, 41]

Cost of nosocomial infections

HAI studies very rarely describe actual costs in money terms but more often they measure the economic impact in terms of proxies, *e.g.* increased length of hospital stay. Even here, the study methodologies vary considerably. A global estimate of this type is that 40 million hospital-days are spent every year due to HAIs.[13] However, measuring the economic impact of HAIs should go beyond the proxy of excess hospitalisation. This was realised as far back as in 1977 when a comprehensive approach to cost analysis of HAIs was defined: "Direct cost is the cost to the health services in terms of health manpower, materials, equipment and facilities. Indirect cost would include the consequences of HAIs on the affected person, on his productivity and services to the community, and therefore on the economy as a whole".[42]

In reality, however, very few cost-estimates of HAIs actually consider all these elements. One method of evaluating cost currently gaining popularity is the Appropriateness Evaluation Protocol (AEP) which seems to compensate for most of the limitations of traditional proxy methods. Appropriateness Evaluation Protocol is diagnosis-independent and is therefore thought to be more objective.[43] The AEP assumes that all information justifying use of in-patient services is contained in the medical record. This information can be divided into three categories:
– original causes of hospitalisation;
– nosocomial infection;
– information related to both original causes and nosocomial infection.

These categories are used to determine whether each day of stay can be justified clinically by one of them.

Previously, the main methodologies used to calculate the cost of HAI were: *a)* comparisons of costs between infected and uninfected patients; *b)* direct physician assessment; and *c)* matched analysis. All three methodologies have their respective advantages and disadvantages,[44] yet common for all three is their infrequent inclusion of indirect costs – especially those incurred after the hospitalisation period. Examples of indirect costs could be: absence from work, home care, rehabilitative measures, income maintenance programmes, social security, etc.

Despite the awareness (for many years now) of the need for a more comprehensive view in estimating total costs of HAIs, few studies have attempted to comply with this approach. This is perhaps due to the cumbersome and difficult efforts required in identifying the needed information. Many countries do, however, have budgetary systems and mechanisms for identifying patients that would allow compilation of cost data from both health care and social institutions, and including periods of hospitalisation and subsequent ambulatory care. It is necessary to consider the indirect costs when calculating global figures on the real impact that HAIs have on the health care system: it cannot be stressed enough that it must be the total cost that is important also when evaluating the cost-benefit of implementing preventive programmes.

It has been stated that no economic evaluation method yet exists that approximates the absolute value of economic consequences of HAIs either overall or for specific sub-sets.[44] This fact stated in 1981 still holds true today and is one of the more pertinent issues in this field in the 1990s.

One exception to the multitude of studies only looking at the hospitalisation period is a French study from 1982 in which 512 patients who underwent gastrointestinal surgery were followed for six months.[45] In this population the number of working days lost due to nosocomial infections was calculated to be 13.8 of which only 3.4 fell during the hospitalisation period. Looking at the convalescence period and trying also to estimate social costs, the authors drew the conclusion that the financial burden of NIs falls largely on the social security budget rather than on the hospital budget. This fact alone should incite third-party payers actively to promote prevention of NI.

Many more studies of this type should be conducted to obtain valid estimates of what NIs "really cost" and better to indicate which budgets are being burdened. The proportion of the total costs not covered by the health care budget will vary according to the financing system, but there seems no doubt that calculating only hospital cost is grossly misleading with regard to the magnitude of the problem.

The economic consequences of HAIs is an area where international collaboration is needed. Assessing cost-benefit in infection control has received much attention, but virtually no change of strategy has occurred at the national level.

The thumb-rule often used is to double the mean length of stay if a hospital infection is acquired. This has proven to be too crude a way to address such a complex problem. In reality, added length of stay depends on several factors, of which the type of infection is the single most important. For example, a urinary tract infection can be effectively treated with a short prolongation of stay, whereas serious surgical wound and blood stream infections can multiply hospital days by as many as 10 times! In addition, the actual method of determining extra length of stay has a great influence on total cost calculation.

In one study, when extra bed days due to infection were determined by physician assessment, these were evaluated to be five days on average. Matched analysis for specific types of patients, when adjusted for case mix, produced an estimate of about 13 additional days. Direct comparisons of infected – with uninfected – controls have given even longer added durations of stay.[46]

Logically, one would expect that extra hospitalisation due to infection was exclusively determined by the type and severity of the infection; valid estimates seem difficult to obtain, however. In a well conducted study of surgical wound infections undertaken in Canada between 1967 and 1977, SWIs were found to have imposed an extra 10 days of hospital stay.[47]

Different incentives also exist in the health care systems for keeping patients with HAIs in hospital or discharging them. This poses an added uncertainty in cost evaluation. In countries where hospitals are paid on a fee-for-service basis, patients will generally be discharged at a quicker pace while in hospitals reimbursed on the basis of occupancy and load factor indicators, perverse incentives exist which may result in the average length of stay for similar procedures being twice as long. This is clearly illustrated when comparing average lengths of stay between US hospitals and German hospitals, with the latter group experiencing double the length of stay.[48]

Despite these difficulties, many attempts have been made to put direct figures on the cost of HAIs. While these are only estimates due to the reasons mentioned above, they serve as "eye openers".

Cost figures of HAIs

In estimates based on a 5% infection rate and an average of four extra days of hospitalisation per patient infected, extrapolation of 1986 figures show that, in that year alone, the overall cost of HAIs to the British National Health Service would have been a loss of 950 000 bed days and £111 million.[49] For Germany, the total estimated added cost due to HAIs in 1984 was DM 500 million to 1 000 million.[50]

Large national extrapolations estimate that 11.5 million extra bed days may be lost in the United States due to HAIs: an annual cost of US$ 1 billion in 1980.[46] For a theoretically-average 250-bed hospital, the annual excess cost due to HAIs is US$ 800 000. It is estimated that this could be reduced by about one-third, if effective infection control programmes were implemented.[51]

When studying added cost by specific procedure, infection following appendectomy increased length of stay by six days and incurred an added cost of US$ 688. Corresponding 1977 figures for caesarian sections were 5.8 days and US$ 527, while for colon resection it was estimated at 13.8 days and US$ 1 591.[52]

More recent publications from Sweden calculate the average length of stay for surgical patients without complications to be 7 days, and up to 12 days when complications occurred. The excess cost per patient in 1989 was estimated at SKr 14 400.[11]

In a 1989 study of coronary artery by-pass surgery, SWIs changed the mean duration of hospitalisation from 8.3 to 26.8 days, and the cost from between US$ 12 000 to 25 000. The net loss to the hospital per infected patient was approximately US$ 2 000, compared with a US$ 3 000 gain if the patient was not infected.[53]

Studying specific patient types in more detail is an approach more frequently carried out today. Such specific studies illustrate more effectively the magnitude of economic consequences due to HAIs rather than crude estimates of mixed patient populations.

Comprehensive longitudinal studies related to cost – including hospitalisation and ambulatory period – are still needed and would be a worthwhile initiative for international collaboration.

Strategies for reducing hospital-acquired infections

Approximately one-third of all HAIs are potentially preventable by means of stringent, effective control programmes.

The most detailed knowledge concerning the efficacy of infection control programmes comes from an American Study on the Efficacy of Nosocomial Infection Control (SENIC) which was carried out over a one-year period during the mid-1970s.[9] This study was co-ordinated by the hospital infection programme of the Centre for Disease Control, Atlanta. The novelty of the SENIC data was that they allowed measurement of the preventive effect of HAIs in relation to surveillance activities, intensity of the infection control effort, teaching activities and overall policy development. One of the important features studied was whether the hospitals regularly provided feedback to surgeons on rates of SWIs.

The study results showed that an overall 32% reduction in HAIs was obtained in participating hospitals where all essential components of intensive infection control programmes were practised. These included:

- Conducting concurrent overall surveillance and control activities;
- presence of a trained infection control physician;
- staffing of one infection control nurse per 250 beds;
- a reporting system for wound infection rates to practising surgeons.

Since only a few hospitals exercised all areas of this programme, it was estimated that 6% of the HAIs were actually being prevented by the mid-1970s, leaving another 26% to be prevented if there were universal adoption of the total SENIC programme.

The authors of the SENIC study calculated that a reduction of only 6.3% in excess hospitalisation would make the infection control programme balance economically. There can be no doubt, therefore, that the introduction of the most stringent prevention strategies would be highly cost-effective.

An update of the SENIC project in 1983 showed that the intensity of infection surveillance and control activities had greatly increased since 1976 in a random sample of hospitals. There had been a large increase in the number of hospitals employing infection control nurses and infection control physicians. These two categories of extra personnel have continuously shown that they are a cost-effective investment, both in United States and in Europe. The improvement in infections in the SENIC update was in selective areas such as prevention of urinary tract infection, bacteraemias and nosocomial pneumonias. These are typically the areas where the impact of the work of infection control nurses would be anticipated.

Unfortunately there was no improvement for SWIs. It was noted that the percentage of hospitals performing continuous SWI surveillance had actually decreased, and the number of hospitals recording surgeon-specific infection rates had fallen from 19 to 13%.[54] This seems particularly unfortunate as SWI surveillance, with feedback to surgeons, is the one strategy repeatedly highlighted as exemplary in terms of effective impact. It is also the one area where the activities of infection control nurses will be the least effective. Surgical wound infections will only decrease when the surgeons commit themselves to the task.

When discussing methods for reducing HAIs, abundant literature exists on a multitude of different procedures. In this kaleidoscopic picture, it is advisable to divide the methods into those that have been scientifically verified and those whose benefits still require further investigation. Verified procedures include:

- sterilisation;
- disinfection;
- handwashing;
- utilisation of closed urinary drainage systems;
- antibiotic prophylaxis for certain types of clean-contaminated and contaminated procedures.

With reference to many other widely used preventive procedures, considerable uncertainty remains regarding which of these practices are truly effective or which are simply used as a matter of tradition or routine.

It is clear that significant cost reduction would be incurred by dispensing with unproven preventive action. This might, by itself, release the necessary funds for introducing validated preventive measures.

Priorities: surgical wound infections

SWIs have been described earlier as the main cause for extra bed days (60%) and the most costly element of HAIs (40%). It is therefore sensible to direct primary efforts towards preventing SWIs.

To prevent SWIs most effectively, the strategy must be multi-faceted and will require a multi-disciplinary approach. Overall effectiveness will largely depend on the openness of the health care personnel to changes in behaviour and adoption of new attitudes, as well as willingness to eliminate traditional "territorial" barriers. However, in addition to psychological and educational approaches, a series of recommendations do exist to reduce SWIs:

a) Instituting a continuous surveillance programme with feedback to surgeons on individual and ward-specific rates;
b) minimising the duration of preoperative stay;
c) minimising the duration of surgery;
d) appropriate use of preoperative prophylactic antibiotics;
e) maintenance of a verified sterile and disinfected environment;
f) use of verified patient preparation methodologies;
g) optimising patients' preoperative conditions (e.g. reduction of obesity, increased physical fitness, improved nutritional status);
h) minimisation of invasive surgery when alternatives exist.

The single most important factor for SWI reduction is the institution of routine surveillance systems which provide timely feedback to surgeons on infection rates.

It has been shown through numerous studies that if surveillance is effectively performed and feedback provided to surgeons, a reduction of 30-50% can be obtained in the incidence of SWIs.[55] This strategy, unfortunately, is not routinely introduced as yet, despite the fact that the classical work of Cruse dates back to 1982. A total of 62 933 wounds were inspected in this study. Definitions of wound infections were standardized, and surveillance was continued by telephone up to 28 days post-operatively. By using this approach, 2 960 wound infections were identified and the overall wound infection rate established at 4.7%. Each surgeon participating in the study received reports showing the individual rates of infection in clean wounds as well as the average clean wound infection rate of the other surgeons in corresponding surgical divisions. Monthly reports of the infection rates were discussed at meetings by the surgical department as well as by the local infection control committee. The result of this effort was a reduction of almost 50% in the overall wound infection rate six months following the introduction of the feedback mechanism.[47]

Similar studies carried out in the late 1980s in Sweden and Denmark have confirmed these results. There is little doubt therefore that periodic feedback to surgeons has a beneficial effect on the rates of SWIs, although the direct causality cannot be established.[56, 57]

In a more recent calculation from Denmark which uses 1986 data, it is estimated that of the 520 000 operative procedures performed, 24 000 SWIs will occur and occupy 300 000 extra bed days. Based on a 20 % reduction of SWIs, this would allow another 7 500 new patients to be operated on per year[58] – an important factor when considering the constant increase in waiting time for non-acute operations. This clearly illustrates that even a minor reduction in SWIs and its consequence on occupancy of beds will have a considerable impact on waiting lists.

In 1987, the Danish National Board of Health recommended that standardized feedback to surgeons on procedure-specific infection rates should be established as a routine.[59] At that time, it was estimated that this practice was only carried out on a regular basis in less than 10-15% of all surgical departments. The initial reluctance by the surgeons to undertake this type of surveillance was most likely due to an inherent resistance amongst surgeons to have rates available which might potentially allow inter-institutional and inter-surgeon comparisons. The situation has changed for the better in more recent years and surgical societies are now becoming more interested in surveillance with feedback; they are actively implementing standardized feedback systems. The percentage of surgical wards undertaking surveillance in Denmark in a standardized format has risen to around 60% in 1990. In addition, a central database has been established at the National Centre of Hygiene, *Statens Seruminstitute,* Copenhagen, to which individual centres are invited to supply aggregated data biannually. This practice has recently been initiated; the preliminary results are promising, however, and will allow the participating centres to see their own results in a larger perspective.

Information systems and HAI prevention

The collection, retrieval, analysis and display of data related to SWIs in a standardized and comprehensive form has been greatly facilitated by the advent of modern information technology. Computerised surveillance, with micro-computer programmes, has proven an effective and feasible way to undertake this task. Creating a monthly infection rate report (including all types of NIs) has been estimated to require a minimum of 20 hours of work per week for a 250-bed hospital. The extra man-hours needed in a surgical department for continuous SWI surveillance is probably much less. Therefore, the classic argument of lack of manpower does not seem valid when considering the potential benefits. Many specific software programmes for this purpose exist or are currently being developed.

A 1988 survey, carried out by the World Health Organisation Regional Office for Europe (WHO/EURO) involved issuance of a simple software to 30 surgical departments in eleven European countries. This study showed that it was possible to obtain data on surgical wound surveillance even from centres with no previous surveillance and/or computer experience.[60] Based on this positive experience a simple non-commercial software, WHOCARE, has been issued by WHO/EURO in collaboration with the Belgian Ministry of Health. On an international scale, the aggregation of SWI data has been facilitated by the distribution of the WHOCARE software which now has a user-network of more than 150 centres, mostly in Europe.[61] Several other similar information systems exist, for example AICE (United States), EPINOSO (France), and IDEAS from the Centre for Disease Control, Atlanta, United States.

Information systems are important tools in obtaining valid data suitable for comparative purposes because they permit data to be collected in a standardized manner. Apart from the positive effects of introducing a surveillance system in individual centres, such a tool allows voluntary aggregation of data for comparative purposes.

HAIs: An indicator of quality of care

During the recent shift in emphasis towards outcome-related indicators, HAI rates have been included in most hospital quality assurance programmes. There are two important reasons for this: first and foremost, a large amount of knowledge exists regarding differences in infection rates; and secondly, effective measures for reducing HAI rates already exist, making this area a relevant starting point for interventional quality assurance programmes.

Using HAIs as one of the indicators of quality has also been promoted by the fact that earlier outcome-related indicators have tended to apply to only a minor proportion of hospitalised patients. Such indicators have included: maternal mortality, peri-operative deaths, deaths during anaesthesia, etc. Death during an operation is fortunately a rare event and therefore monitoring of such incidents cannot be used as a proxy for the general quality of hospital care. HAIs provide a better proxy for evaluating general quality, although they should not carry the burden alone. Efforts are currently being made to compile a series of outcome-related indicators which may collectively measure the quality of hospital services.

Areas of focus for the 1990s

A prerequisite for advancing in the area of HAI prevention is recognition that the issue should no longer be seen as a purely medical problem. Greater awareness must be created, emphasizing that HAIs are also a social, political and economic problem of great magnitude – one where there is considerable potential for rapid improvement.

In an attempt to identify the areas of specific focus listed below, it became clear that some areas relate to already well-established strategies with known benefit, while others relate to areas where more research is needed to direct future preventive programmes:

- introduction of continuous surveillance systems producing specific feedback for surgeons on infection rates;
- detailed cost-effectiveness studies of a longitudinal nature, to investigate costs incurred in and out of hospital in relation to infection control strategies;
- policy formulation and, more importantly, implementation and adherence to rational antibiotic use;
- adoption of verified infection-surveillance strategies in hospitals, as well as abandonment of obsolete practices;
- definition of specific patient risk groups towards which infection prevention programmes are directed;
- analysis of the changing use of existing technologies and emergence of new technologies with respect to their effect on HAI rates, especially the use of intravascular devices.

In conclusion....

From the previous overview of the occurrence and cost of HAIs, it should be plain that there already exists an abundance of available data and analyses on the subject. Continuing duplication of incidence and prevalence studies should no longer top the list of priorities. Rather, the 1990s should be the decade of dissemination of knowledge, the time to implement those strategies which have already been verified, and which are known to reduce and prevent HAIs.

To ensure this process, a multi-disciplinary approach will be necessary, as well as an openness and willingness on the part of health care professionals to commit themselves to the task.

Obviously, the level of advancement in HAI prevention strategies varies from centre to centre, from country to country. The expertise of local specialists should be used wherever possible to tailor the needs of each individual institution.

Hospital management must supply the encouragement and show a positive attitude, which is the crucial element of success in any health care programme.

Commitment on the part of policy-makers and health economists at local, national and international levels is also needed.

And finally, it bears repeating that, although no strategy can be perfectly delineated to fit all institutions, top priority should nonetheless be given to the implementation of specific surgical surveillance and feedback reports which provide doctors themselves with HAI rates. Here is a practice which can be instituted immediately, a strategy which has repeatedly produced a positive benefit.

We have the tools to do something about HAIs.

What is needed is the will to use them.

Bibliographical notes

1. Vuor, H.V. (1982), "Quality assurance of health services", *Public Health in Europe,* WHO Regional Office for Europe, No. 16, Copenhagen.

2. Donabedian, A. (1966), "Evaluating the quality of medical care", *The Milbank Memorial Fund Quarterly,* 44:166-206.

3. World Health Organisation (1989), Monitoring of the strategy for health for all by the year 2000. Part 1: *The situation in the European region, 1987/1988;* Part 2: *Monitoring by country, 1988/1989,* WHO Regional Office for Europe, Copenhagen.

4. Retinopathy Working Party (1991), "A protocol for screening for diabetic retinopathy in Europe", *Diabetic Medicine,* 8:263-7.

5. Department of Health (1989), *Report on confidential enquiries into maternal deaths in England and Wales 1982-84,* London, HMSO.

6. Berwick, DM. (1989), "Continuous improvement as an ideal in health care", *New England Journal of Medicine,* 320:53-6.

7. Moss, F. (1992), "Quality in health care", *Quality in Health Care,* 1:1-3.

8. Worning, A.M. (1991), "Hospital acquired infections. The size of the problem. Strategies for reduction", an OECD Working Paper (unpublished).

9. Haley, R. W., Culyer, D.H., and White, J.W. (1985), "The efficacy of infection surveillance and control programs in preventing nosocomial infections in US hospitals", *American Journal of Epidemiology,* 121:182-305.

10. Elandt-Johnson, R.C. (1975), "Definition of rates: some remarks on their use and misuse", *American Journal of Epidemiology,* 102(4):267-71.

11. SPRI (1990), Kvalitetssäkring i kirurgi och anestesiologi. SPRI Report 289, Stockholm, The Swedish Planning and Rationalization Institute for Health and Social Services.

12. Reimer, K., Gleed, C. and Nicolle, L.E. (1983), "The impact of postdischarge infection on surgical wound infection rates", *Infection Control,* 11:226-9.

13. Sabri, S. and Tittensor, J.R. (1982), *Hospital infection and its control,* Proceedings of the first Middle East Symposium, Kuwait 1981, Barker Publications, Surrey.

14. Jepsen, O.B. and Mortensen, N. (1980), "Prevalence of nosocomial infection and infection control in Denmark", *Journal on Hospital Infection,* 1:237-44.

15. Hovig, B. *et al.* (1981), "A prevalence survey of infections among hospitalized patients in Norway", *NIPH Ann,* 4(2):49-60.

16. Moro, M.L. *et al.* (1986), "National prevalence survey of hospital-acquired infections in Italy, *Journal of Hospital Infection,* 8:72-85.

17. Danchaivijitr, S. and Waitayapiches, S. (1988), "Prevalence of nosocomial infections in Siriraj Hospital 1983-1986", *J Med Assoc Thailand,* 71 (supplement 3):5-10.

18. Mertens, R. *et al.* (1987), "The national prevalence survey of nosocomial infections in Belgium, 1984", *Journal of Hospital Infection,* 9:219-29.

19. Maderova, E. *et al.* (1987), "Prevalence of nosocomial infections in selected hospitals", *Journal of Hyg Epidemiol Immunol,* 31(4):365-74.

20. McLaws, M.L. (1988), "The prevalence of nosocomial and community-acquired infections in Australian hospitals", *Medical Journal of Australia,* 149:582-90.

21. Sramova, H. *et al.* (1988), "National prevalence survey of hospital-acquired infections in Czechoslovakia", *Journal of Hospital Infection,* 11:328-34.

22. Dancaivijitr, S. and Chokloikaew, S. (1989), "A national prevalence study on nosocomial infections 1988" *Journal Med Assoc Thailand,* 72 (suppl.2):1-6.

23. EPINE (1990), *Prevalencia de las infecciones nosocomiales en los hospitales españoles*, Sociedad española de higiene y medicina preventiva hospitalarias y grupo de trabajo epincat.

24. Jepsen, O.B., Olesen-Larsen, S. and Dankert, J. *et al.* (1982), "Urinary tract infection and bacteremia in hospitalized medical patients – a European multicentre prevalence survey on nosocomial infections", *Journal of Hospital Infection,* 3:241-52.

25. Manyon-White, R.T. *et al.* (1988), "An international survey of the prevalence of hospital-acquired infections", *Journal of Hospital Infection,* (Suppl. A) : 43-8.

26. EURO-NIs (1991), "Nosocomial infections and health care practices in intensive care units in Europe", Result of Survey A (second analysis) of 1 005 intensive care units, EEC EURO-NIs Project, COMAC HSR, Institut d'Épidémiologie, Lyon.

27. Green, J.W. and Wenzel, R.P. (1977), "Postoperative wound infection: a controlled study of the increased duration of hospital stay and direct cost of hospitalization", *Ann Surg,* 185(3):264-8.

28. Bunt, T.J. (1983), "Synthetic vascular graft infections; clinical review", *Surgery,* 93:733-45.

29. Fitzgerald, R.H.Jr. (1989), "Infections of hip prostheses and artificial joints", *Infect Dis Clin North Am,* 3:329-38.

30. Rand, J.A. and Fitzgerald, R.H.Jr. (1989), "Diagnosis and management of the infected total knee arthroplasty", *Orthop Clin North Am,* 20:201-10.

31. Bartlett, J.G., O'Keefe, P., Tally, F.P. *et al.* (1986), "Bacteriology of hospital-acquired pneumonia", *Arch Intern Med,* 146:868-71.

32. Fagon, J.-Y., Chastre, J., and Domart, Y. (1989), "Nosocomial pneumonia in patients receiving continuous mechanical ventilation", *American Review Resp Dis,* 139:877-84.

33. Hamory, B.H. (1987), Nosocomial bloodstream and intravascular device-related infections, in Wenzel, R.P. (ed), *Prevention and control of nosocomial infections,* Williams & Wilkins, Baltimore: 283-319.

34. Maki, D.G. and Will, L. (1990), "Risk factors for central venous catheter-related infections within the ICU. A prospective study of 345 catheters", 3rd Decennial International Conference on Nosocomial Infections, Atlanta, Georgia, July 3l-August 3, Abstract No. 54.

35. Burke, J.F. (1961), "The effective period of preventive antibiotic action in experimental incisions and dermal lesions", *Surgery,* 50:161-8.

36. Swedish Board of Health (1984), *Antibiotics and Surgery,* National Board of Health and Welfare Drug Information Committee, Uppsala, Sweden.

37. NSIH – Protocole d'étude, Phase pilote October-December 1991, Programme national pour la surveillance des infections hospitalières.

38. "Antibiotic use and antibiotic resistance worldwide" (1987), *Reviews of Infectious Diseases,* Vol. 9, suppl. 3, May-June.

39. Staehr, Johansen K. *et al.* (1988), "An international study on the occurrence of multiresistant bacteria and aminoglycoside patterns", *Infection,* 16:(5):313-22.

40. Marr, J.J., Moffet, H.L. and Kunin, C.M. (1988), "Guidelines for improving the use of antimicrobial agents in hospitals: a statement by the Infectious Diseases Society of America", *J Infect Dis,* 157:869-76.

41. Kunin, C.M., Staehr Johansen K., Worning, A.M. and Daschner, F.D. (1990), "Report of a Symposium on Use and Abuse of Antibiotics Worldwide", *Rev Infect Dis,* 12(1):12-19.

42. Wahba, A.H.W. (1977), "Economic aspects of hospital infections", Presentation made at the International Workshop on proven and unproven methods in hospital infection control, Baiersbronn, 24-25 September (unpublished document), WHO Regional Office for Europe, Copenhagen.

43. Wakefield, D.S., and Pfaller, M. (1992), "Methods for Estimating Days of Hospitalization Due to Nosocomial Infections", *Medical Care,* 30(4):373-76.

44. McGowan, J.E. (1981), "Cost and benefit in control of nosocomial infection: methods for analysis", *Rev Infect Dis,* 3(4)-790-7.

45. Fabry, J., Meynet, R., and Joron, M.T. (1982), "Cost of Nosocomial Infections: Analysis of 512 Digestive Surgery Patients", *World Journal of Surgery,* 6:362-65.

46. Haley, R.W. *et al.* (1985), "Estimating the extra charges and prolongation of hospitalization due to nosocomial infections: a comparison of methods", *Journal of Infect Dis,* 141(2):248-57.

47. Cruse, P.J.E. and Foord, R. (1980), "The epidemiology of wound infection. A 10 year prospective study of 62 939 wounds'", *Surg Clin North Am,* 60(1):27-40.

48. Daschner, F.D. (1989), "Cost-effectiveness in hospital infection control lessons for the 1990s", *Journal of Hospital Infection,* 1989, 13:325-36.

49. Currie, E. and Maynard, A. (1989), "Economic Aspects of Hospital Acquired Infection", Discussion Paper 56, Centre for Health Economics, University of York, York, June.

50. Dashner, F.D. (1984), "The cost of hospital-acquired infection", *Journal of Hospital Infection*, 5 (Suppl. A) : 27-33.

51. Dixon, R.E. (1987), "Costs of nosocomial infections and benefits of infection control programs", in: *Prevention and Control of Nosocomial Infections*, Wenzel, R.P. Williams and Wilkins (*ed.*), Baltimore.

52. Green, J.W. and Wenzel, R.P. (1977), "Postoperative wound infection: a controlled study of the increased duration of hospital stay and direct cost of hospitalization", *Ann Surg*, 185(3):264-8.

53. Taylor, G.J., Mikell, F.L., Moses, H.W. (1990), "Determinants of hospital charges for coronary artery bypass surgery: the economic consequences of postoperative complications", *American Journal of Cardiology*, 65(5): 309-13.

54. Haley, R.W., Morgan, W.M., Culver, D.H., White, J.W. (1985), "Hospital infection control: Recent progress and opportunities under prospective payment", *Am. J Infect. Control*, 13:97-107.

55. Olson, M., O'Connor, M. and Schwartz, M. (1984), "Surgical wound infections. A 5-year prospective study of 20,193 wounds at the Minneapolis VA Medical Center", *Ann Surg*, 199:253-9.

56. Sejberg, D. *et al.* (1989), "Postoperative saarinfektioner paa en blandet kirurgisks afdeling", *Vidensab og Praksis*, 991-4.

57. Kjellgren, K., *et al.* (1985), "Registrering avkirurgiska infectioner kan 'spara' mangmiljonbelopp i varden", *Läkartidningen*, 82:4428-31.

58. Jepsen, O.B. (1990), "Infektioner efter operationer sluger sengedage", *Journal 2*, National Board of Health publication, Denmark.

59. "Raad & anvisninger om registrering af postoperative saarinfektioner. Den centrale afd. for sygehushygiejne" (1988), Statens Seruminstitut.

60. "Developing quality of care through information systems: hospital infection surveillance as a model" (1990), Report on a WHO Workshop, Copenhagen, 26-28 April 1989. Doc. ref. EUR/ICP/CLR 049, World Health Organization, Regional Office for Europe, Copenhagen.

61. Staehr Johansen, K. (1992), "WHOCARE: hospital infection surveillance and feedback programme", in *Current perspectives in healthcare computing 1992*, Proceedings of a Conference held in Harrogate, 9-11 March, *The British Journal of Healthcare Computing*, Surrey.

QUALITY OF CARE AND THE REFORM AGENDA
IN THE ACUTE HOSPITAL SECTOR

by

Miriam M. Wiley

Introduction

"(...) The more aggressive cost-containing atmosphere of the PPS (Prospective Payment System) was not accompanied by a cost-quality trade-off (...). The forces that push up health care costs will probably not abate in the near future, but one possible lesson from the PPS experience is that we can simultaneously contain costs and improve quality" (Wilensky, 1990).

An issue of importance for international developments in the health care field is placed centre stage here, and the question which must be asked is whether there is evidence to support the view that quality of care will inevitably suffer in an environment of cost control. The continued paucity of information at both the national level and the international level means that we are still not in a position to give a definitive answer to this question here. Our objective, instead, is to consolidate the available evidence for selected OECD countries so that the current stage of evolution of the cost/quality dichotomy may be assessed on a more informed basis.

The comment by Wilensky noted above was made in association with the publication of a study by the RAND corporation on the effects on quality of the reimbursement reform for hospital care under the Prospective Payment System (PPS). While specific findings emerging from this study will be discussed in more detail below, it may be helpful to indicate here that, at its most conservative, the results may be interpreted as indicating that the introduction of PPS has not been associated with a "worsening of outcome" for hospitalised Medicare patients (Kahn *et al.,* 1990, p. 1984). Most optimistically, Rubenstein *et al.* (1990) conclude that "the quality of medical care improved after the introduction of the PPS should serve as encouraging news – hospitals, physicians, and other health professionals continue to put patient need first".

In providing concrete evidence to inform the debate on the nature of the relationship between quality of care and cost control, this study also moves the debate to a more sophisticated plane of analysis. This view is strongly supported by Russell (1989) who also undertook a study of the effects of the US PPS and concluded that it has been associated with a "new concern with quality (...). Until 1983 quality was largely taken for granted (...). Now that quality is recognised as something that will not take care of itself, data systems and review mechanisms must be developed to monitor, measure, and encourage its existence" (pp. 85-86).

The view emerging from these studies is that the reform of reimbursement for hospital services in an environment of cost control has been associated with establishing a place for quality assessment and enhancement on the permanent health care agenda. Moving beyond the United States on to the international platform, it is apparent that there is a generalised absence of data on the nature of the relationship between cost control policies and quality of care. What is encountered, however, is a trend towards the implementation of proposals for reform of financing/funding arrangements for acute hospital services. Given the current stage of development of these reforms, the furthest an assessment of the question posed at the outset can go in the international context is to enquire if quality concerns are part of the same agenda as the financing reforms and, if so, what form does this agenda item take?

The concept of "quality" may appear to have chameleon-like characteristics at times – the ability to adapt to the shape and appearance of the surrounding environment. A detailed assessment of approaches to the measurement of quality would, however, warrant a complete document in itself. The focus here, therefore, concentrates on a specific theoretical dimension which has come to the fore in more recent studies of quality assessment. This concerns the issue of standardization for patient-type which is common to both financing reform and quality assessment. An assessment of proposals for such reform in a number of countries follows and this review concludes with an assessment of the dominant trends emerging, with particular reference to the cost/quality dichotomy.

Quality assessment and case-mix measurement

While there is general agreement that any attempt to measure quality of care must be multidimensional, there is less agreement about the precise nature of the model which should be applied. Perhaps the most widely reported model in the literature may be traced back to Donabedian (1966), who identified three approaches to the assessment of quality: structure, process and outcome. While there are inter-relationships among these approaches, the development of operational measures of quality have tended to be limited rather than comprehensive.

The incorporation of the outcome dimension, in particular, into a more broadly integrated model of quality assessment had to await the 1960s, though documented attempts to measure patients' outcomes predates this departure by several decades. In the celebrated and frequently cited work of Codman (1914, 1916) there is evidence of early efforts systematically to record information relating to patient care outcomes. Codman's contribution is as significant for its recognition of the deficiencies of the tools at his disposal, as for his innovative approach to information collection and analysis. A core problem identified by Codman as a serious constraint hampering his research was the absence of a standardized definition of the hospital product which could be used as a framework for assessment of quality (Codman, 1914).

Any serious attempts to address this very fundamental problem had to await the 1960s and 1970s and the technology which could tackle the large data bases required to standardized the definition of the hospital product. To a great extent, it was the challenge presented by this objective which sparked initial interest in the growth of an area of research focusing on the development of case-mix measures for hospital care.

The implication that case-mix definition is necessary for quality assessment arises from the following definitions proposed by Hornbrook (1985): *case-mix* is "the proportion of cases of each disease and health problem treated in the hospital" (p. 296); and *quality* is "the hospital's contribution to the successful outcome or resolution of patients' illnesses or health problems" (p. 295). The case-mix/quality relationship is clearly located along the outcome dimension by Hornbrook.

The nature of the relationship between case-mix measurement and quality assessment is further clarified by Donabedian as follows:

"The purpose of adjustment for differences in case-mix is to reveal the true effects of differences in quality by reducing, as much as possible, the confounding effects of other factors" (Donabedian, 1987, p. 78).

Support for this perspective is forthcoming from a number of sources, including a report on the "Case-Mix Measurement and Assessing Quality of Hospital Care" symposium, published in the 1987 *Health Care Financing Review*. While the symposium aired a wide range of views on many issues, only those contributions relevant to the relationship between quality and case-mix adjustment will be noted here:

"Case-mix adjustment is clearly essential in assessments of the quality of care, whether of secular trends, of the comparative utility of competing patient management techniques, or of the comparative performance of hospitals" (Krakauer, 1987, p. 46).

"If one chooses to measure patient satisfaction or outcome of care, then adjustment for differences in case-mix must be made in order to make a definitive statement about the impact of a structural measure, such as the hospital, on quality of care" (Brook, 1987, p. 43).

The theoretical basis for an integral relationship between measures of case-mix and quality has therefore been strongly supported by recent research on this question. Our specific interest in this contribution will be to review recent initiatives in a number of OECD countries which have identified case-mix measurement and quality assessment as important components of a comprehensive drive to improve the efficiency and effectiveness of performance of the acute hospital sector.

This review must, of necessity, commence with a brief description of the case-mix measurement approach. This will be followed by a synopsis of the most widespread application and evaluation of case-mix adjustment and quality assurance within a hospital programme, *i.e.* the US prospective payment system (PPS). The range of responses to the same issues will then be reviewed on the basis of recent reports from a number of European countries and Australia.

Case-mix measurement

A case-mix classification scheme may be described as a framework which "provides a means for examining the products of the hospital, since patients within each class are expected to receive a similar product" (Fetter *et al.*, 1980). A number of different classification schemes have been developed for the hospital in-patient sector in pursuit of this objective. The recently developed schemes include the Diagnosis-Related Groups (DRG), Medisgroups, Disease Staging, Computerised Severity Index, APACHE II, and Patient Management Categories. While a review of the full range of available schemes is beyond the scope of this contribution, it is relevant to note that these schemes have provided the basis for a number of important comparative studies. The conclusion emerging from one such study undertaken by the Prospective Payment Commission in the United States (1988) is that "diagnosis-related groups (DRGs) are the most appropriate available measure of hospital case-mix for PPS" (p. 3). A few European experts prefer, however, other classifications.

While Disease Staging and Patient Management Categories are the subject of experimentation in a number of European countries, the DRG system is now the most widely used case-mix classification scheme in Australia, Europe, and the United States. Without getting into the mechanics of the system, the essence of the DRG approach may be summarised as identifying in the acute care sector "a set of case types, each representing a class of patients with similar processes of care and a predictable package of services (or product) from an institution" (Fetter, *et al.*, 1981, (p. 27). In excess of 470 DRGs have been defined and more detailed technical information on the construction of the DRG system may be found in a number of sources, including Fetter *et al.* (1980) and Wiley and Fetter (1990).

The fact that standardization is one of the primary attractions of case-mix classification has already been noted above. As a means of illustrating the facility for standardization which the DRG system offers, Table 1 presents data on average length of stay (ALOS) for selected high-volume DRGs for a number of OECD Member countries for 1988. In presenting these data, it must be recognised at the outset that length of stay is an output measure, not an outcome measure. ALOS may also offer a reasonable proxy for resource use as studies have shown high correlations with patient charges (Luke, 1979; Lave and Leinhardt, 1976; Hornbrook and Goldfarb, 1981). While ALOS data are therefore of limited relevance for outcome studies, Table 1 illustrates how the application of a case-mix measure like the DRGs enables us to compare management of similar patient types in different countries.

The relevance of the comparisons in Table 1 is greatly enhanced by the fact that they are standardized for the same type of case, with controls for age, sex, complications/comorbidities and discharge status. This may be more fully appreciated by examining in greater detail the treatment of cases of appendicectomy within this framework. If ALOS for this procedure was to be compared across these countries, it would be reasonable to expect that there would be substantial variation. Part of this

Table 1. **Mean length of stays by case-mix – DRG (days), 1988**

	Lens procedures 39	Tonsillectomy/ adenoidectomy 60	Otitis media 70	Chronic pulmonary disorders 88	Bronchitis/asthma 98	Vein ligation and stripping 119
Belgium	6.4	1.9	4.9	14.3	7.0	5.0
Finland	7.1	2.0	2.9	8.6	3.8	3.1
France	8.2	1.8	3.5	11.3	3.8	4.7
Ireland	5.7	6.1	4.9	7.4	4.8	..
New Zealand	4.0	..	2.5	13.6	..	3.7
Norway	4.9	3.1	..	10.1	..	..
Spain	6.5	1.9	3.8	9.7	4.9	6.6
United States	1.3	1.2	2.8	7.2	3.2	3.7

Source: OECD, 1993.

variation could be legitimately attributed to factors like the effect of complications/comorbidities and/or age in the treatment of this condition. To control for these factors, patients with appendicectomy within the DRG system may be subdivided into four groups on the basis of age and the presence/absence of complications or comorbidities. The comparison of ALOS for DRG 167 presented in Table 1 is restricted to those patients who had an appendicectomy without complication, who were aged less than 70 years. Because of standardization for variables which have a significant effect on treatment process and resource use, the information presented in Table 1 may be legitimately offered as cross-national comparisons for similar patient types.

In the absence of cross-national data on outcomes, Table 1 offers a useful example of how the methodology for the assessment of quality might be usefully advanced. If indicators of outcome like readmission rates, or mortality rates, could be substituted for ALOS, then the power of any variation observed would be greatly enhanced by the use of a standardized case-mix framework.

The opportunities offered by this perspective are now being recognised. Indeed, a World Health Organisation (WHO) investigation of this approach led Vuori and Roger (1989) to conclude that:

"The patient classification system of diagnosis-related groups (DRGs) may become a key tool for quality assurance... Provided that similar groups can be developed for out-patients and patients in nursing and long-term care, DRGs can play an important role in quality assurance: they will help to get comparable statistics and to promote joint quality reviews of medically and economically comparable patients" (p. 128).

The review in this and the previous section has shown that approaches to defining and operational-ising the concepts of outcomes and case-mix measurement have advanced considerably in recent years. This article will explore some of the opportunities offered by recent initiatives in hospital financing and management to give effect to the contribution expected from these advancements. While a number of countries have progressed some distance along the road towards the implementation of reforms, similar proposals are under consideration in other systems. It is hoped that the documented effects on quality in those countries where reforms have been put in place, will help to ensure that implementation is on the main agenda for those new to reform. The most advanced reform, the US Prospective Payment System (PPS) will first be considered, followed by a review of developments in other OECD Member states.

The prospective payment system: expenditure control and quality of care

The Prospective Payment System (PPS) which operates within the Medicare programme is proba-bly the most analysed payment reform in the world. As such, it may be expected to provide some of the richest data available on the relationship between financial incentives, uptake of services and quality. When the PPS was introduced in 1983, it was recognised as the most revolutionary change applied to the Medicare programme during its lifetime (Russell, 1989). During Medicare's first sixteen years of operation, hospitals were reimbursed on the basis of actual costs incurred. Since the introduction of PPS, hospitals have been reimbursed on the basis of a prospectively determined payment for a specified product, defined on the basis of the hospital discharge (ProPAC, 1991a).

The objectives guiding the implementation of the PPS were primarily driven by the belief that it offered greater control over hospital costs and predictability of expenditure, in addition to providing incentives towards the improvement of efficiency at the hospital level (Russell, 1989). There was an obvious risk allied with these objectives, however, in that a reduction in hospital costs could also be achieved by limiting the provision of required services and restricting access to care. To guard against this eventuality, the US Congress mandated the establishment of Peer Review Organisations (PROs) to "monitor quality" in conjunction with the implementation of the PPS.

The quality issue therefore occupied an explicit part of the PPS agenda at the outset. An additional control which the US Congress also put in place at the same time involved the establishment of the Prospective Payment Assessment Commission (ProPAC). This commission was charged with the responsibility of examining and evaluating all factors arising in the determination of Medicare payment. ProPAC publishes a number of reports annually with detailed analyses and recommendations on critical issues like payment rates, expenditure levels, case-mix measurement, etc. ProPAC has also reported regularly on quality assessment and highlighted areas of concern.

It is not intended here to review the PPS since its inception. In the introduction, some of the recent findings of studies dedicated to this objective were noted. At the level of analysis targeted by this study, we are more immediately concerned with defining the place assigned to the goal of quality assessment and assurance within the context of a programme originally conceived as a cost-containment initiative. The questions which arise are therefore: to what extent have the multiple objectives of the programme been achieved in eight years of operation? Has expenditure increased or decreased? Have advancements in cost-containment been at the expense of quality? Have advances been recorded in the understanding and operationalising of the objective of "monitoring quality"? The information available to answer these questions will now be reviewed.

Expenditure control under the PPS

The rate of growth of total and in-patient payments under Medicare slowed considerably after the implementation of the PPS. The annual rate of growth in aggregate Medicare in-patient payments dropped from the 17% recorded in the six years prior to PPS to 6.1% in the six years post-PPS. The rate of growth of total Medicare payments also declined substantially, dropping from the 17.8% recorded annually between 1977 and 1983 to the 9.2% annual rate of change recorded between 1983 and 1989. In looking to the future, however, a report from the HCFA (Health Care Financing Administration, 1991) notes with concern the increased rate of growth of Medicare benefit payments for in-patient hospital care in 1988 compared with previous years. This concern is also echoed by ProPAC which, while deriving some encouragement from the direction of the trend in the rate of growth, notes that "hospital costs have continued to increase faster than the prices of the resources hospitals use in providing inpatient care" (ProPAC, 1991a, p. 14).

Another important measure of the effectiveness of the PPS as a cost control programme is to estimate current expenditure levels relative to what would have been expected in the absence of the programme. This is a very useful means of estimating the level of real savings which may be attributed to the introduction of the PPS. This is the approach adopted by Russell (1989) who concludes that prospective payment has succeeded in its primary objective of slowing the growth of Medicare spending and proceeds to estimate that expenditures are now "expected to be $18 billion less in 1990 than was estimated in the early 1980s – a saving of about 20%. Even when extra spending for out-patient care, possibly due to prospective payment, is deducted, the net saving in 1990 is more than $17 billion" (p. 84). It should be noted, however, that the magnitude of the response to the introduction of the PPS may be somewhat biased by anticipatory effects which would have been expected to occur in the year immediately prior to implementation. While it is difficult to quantify these effects and make the necessary adjustment, it seems sufficient for the purpose of this review to recognise that, while the scale of the post-PPS change may warrant a downward adjustment, the direction of the change is not in dispute.

There are no claims in any of the studies reviewed that the financing and funding problems have been solved within the Medicare programme specifically, or the US health-care system generally. More generic problems associated with the financing and organisation of US health service delivery are the subject of ongoing investigation within the research community and debate among policy-makers. The basic structural problems which persist within the delivery system lead Coulam and Gaumer (1992) to comment that "insofar as PPS and PROs are consistent with the fragmented, payer-by-payer micromanagement of health care costs characteristic of current public and private initiatives, the continued growth of US health care expenditures at least supports a speculation that more fundamental reform is needed, even if, standing alone, the direct and measurable effects of PPS point generally to the success of the PPS effort for the Medicare program" (p. 62). While acknowledging the problems which persist, the evidence available to date does, however, indicate that the introduction of PPS has been associated with a greater degree of control over costs than was previously the case. Given the success which must be acknowledged for the PPS in improving cost control, the next question is whether this objective has been achieved at the expense of cut-backs in quality.

Quality and the PPS

In keeping with the multi-faceted nature of the programme, ProPAC examines a range of quality measures in pursuing its mandate to evaluate all factors affected by Medicare payment issues. The core measures reviewed by ProPAC include readmission, transfers, mortality and in-patient utilisation trends for "at risk" patient groups. The findings reported by ProPAC (1990) for these measures may be summarised as follows:

- The average annual change in 30-day readmission rates of plus 2% recorded for 1979-1983 has changed to an annual average of 1.8% between 1986 and 1988;
- While most hospital transfers could be considered quality enhancing, the growth in the transfer rate of approximately 9% annually between 1985 and 1988 warrants further investigation;
- An assessment of 30-day post-admission mortality rates indicates that patient outcomes are better when high volumes of procedures are performed, and that both mortality rates and costs are inversely related to the volume of procedures performed in a hospital;
- The findings for the "at risk" diagnosis groups led ProPAC to conclude that "access to care for the categorically and medically needy beneficiaries appears to be improving over time" and that "it does not appear that PPS has had gross adverse impacts on either access to care or quality of care for these patient groups" (p. 81).

While these findings may, on the whole, be interpreted as a positive reflection on the operation of the post-PPS Medicare programme, the HCFA has gone further in search of objective measures and evaluation of quality. As part of this endeavour, many individual grants have been awarded to researchers to support the pursuit of this objective. Among the most extensive studies on quality is the RAND Corporation's four-year evaluation of the effects of the DRG-based PPS for hospitalised Medicare patients. Key findings from this study published in a series of articles in the *Journal of the American Medical Association* (October 1990) have already been noted above and will now be discussed in more detail.

Using an analysis based on both explicit process criteria and implicit review, the RAND study estimates the effect of the PPS on quality for a specified number of diseases over the 1981-1986 period. The application of explicit process criteria to four medical conditions (congestive heart failure, myocardial infarction, pneumonia, cerebrovascular accident) led Kahn *et al.* (1990*a*) to estimate that:

1. the 24% decrease recorded after the introduction of PPS was not associated with a deterioration in the process of in-hospital care; and
2. that process improvements across these medical conditions were associated with a 1% reduction in 30-day mortality after the introduction of PPS.

The results of the analysis conducted by implicit review are equally encouraging as the summary findings of Rubenstein *et al.* (1990) show that "the quality of hospital care has continued to improve for Medicare patients despite, or because of, the introduction of the prospective payment system" (p. 1974).

An important cautionary note emerges from the RAND study, however. Both sickness at admission and impairment at discharge were examined as a means of developing disease-specific measures of sickness. The "quicker and sicker" charge sometimes levied at PPS on the basis of anecdotal evidence received some support as the proportion of patients discharged home in an unstable condition was found to have increased from the 10 per cent level recorded prior to PPS, to a level of 15 per cent after the implementation of PPS (Kosekoff *et al.*, 1990, p. 1980). This finding must, however, be balanced against the results of the Keeler *et al.* (1990) analysis indicating that sickness level on admission increased following the introduction of PPS, a factor which would have to be taken into account in any assessment of the effects of PPS on mortality level.

Too often there is resistance to the introduction of cost-control policies in the health field, for fear that they will be detrimental to quality. Existing evidence, however, makes a strong case for quite the opposite: namely that implementation of a case-mix based system for determining payment to hospitals on a prospective basis has been associated with:

- cost-containment, and
- quality assurance, indeed enhancement.

This conclusion is supported by Coulam and Gaumer (1992) in their evaluation of the effects of the PPS on the US Medicare system: "PPS appears to have saved Medicare money without causing systematic, documented harm to patients or the health care industry" (p. 72). The remainder of this review will focus on the international community to assess the evidence available for parallel developments in other OECD countries.

International developments

There are no exact replicas of the Medicare hospital reimbursement system outside the United States, so a scientific study of comparative performance on the two factors of expenditure control and quality assurance is not possible. There are, however, some important international initiatives which parallel the PPS in a number of important dimensions. These initiatives will be reviewed here with the aim of identifying any common ground in objectives and/or outcome for these programmes.

The task to this end, therefore, consists in attempting a synthesis of work in progress in selected OECD countries, towards the development of case-mix based applications within their respective health-care systems. The countries included in this review can be differentiated into two groups initially: those concerned primarily with the development of case-mix based applications for financing purposes; and, secondly, those oriented towards the development of planning and management applications.

Those Member countries for which objectives related to financing have been proposed are listed in Table 2. This contribution is not attempting an exhaustive review of the different health systems represented here, or the details of the reforms planned or being implemented (OECD, 1992; OECD, forthcoming). It has therefore been necessary to identify relevant characteristics across which the developments of interest can be assessed. The characteristics presented in Table 2 are concerned with financing descriptors and approaches to case-mix measurement and quality assurance.

While a majority of OECD countries are considering some form of health system reform, the listing presented here has been limited to facilitate a more in-depth analysis of specific proposals. Seven of the countries listed in Table 2, including the United States, are at the point of implementing recommended reforms at some level, while reforms are reported to be in the process of being developed or proposed in the remaining countries. It is interesting to note the consistency across the countries reviewed in terms of a number of descriptors, particularly the time frame, the application of a case-mix measure, and quality assurance/assessment procedures. Regardless of implementation status, all countries report a preference for prospective, rather than retrospective, financing of hospital services. Case-mix measure(s) and quality assurance measure(s) are also proposed, or in use, in association with reforms in the financing of hospitals in these countries. While the approach to quality assurance proposed as part of the reforms varies across countries, there is a high degree of consistency in the type of case-mix measure proposed. For the majority of these countries, the DRG system is the preferred option, with three countries on this list currently in the process of developing national case-mix systems. For a number of countries, there is also the commitment to use, or experiment with, more than one case-mix measure.

With regard to the unit of payment, only the United States has indicated a preference for patient-based payment for hospital services. A global-budget approach is the predominant technique adopted, or proposed, in five of the countries listed here, while the remaining four countries operate within a mixed system. The majority of countries report that funding comes from a number of sources, including government, while government funding is the primary source in the remaining countries. An appreciation of the combined impact of these different indicators demands a more detailed description of the reforms/proposals in these countries; this will now be provided.

Country reform profiles

Australia

The search for improved ways of paying for hospital services has stimulated extensive research in *Australia,* both at the State and the Commonwealth levels (Duckett, 1988; Palmer, 1990). Much of this research has been oriented towards relating hospital reimbursement to an agreed definition of the hospital product. Within this context, there has been widespread experimentation with case-mix classification measures, and particularly the DRG system. The establishment of the Case-Mix Development Programme by the Commonwealth government has resulted in funding being made available for projects concerned with the application of the DRG system to budgeting and planning for hospital service provision, and for the development and implementation of utilisation review and quality assurance programmes. In presenting recommendations arising out of a detailed study of the potential for case payment in Australian hospitals, the authors conclude that:

"It would be undesirable to implement PPS without being able to assess the effects on quality, and we support the principle of encouraging quality assurance within the context of a PPS, for example,

Table 2. **Summary characteristics of financing reform, case-mix classification and quality assurance for selected OECD countries**

	Australia	Belgium	United Kingdom	France	Ireland	Norway	Portugal	Spain	Sweden	United States
Financing reform										
Time frame	Prospective	Prospective	Prospective	Prospective	Prospective	Prospective	Prospective	Prospective	Prospective	Prospective
Unit	Budget	Mixed	Mixed	Mixed	Budget	Mixed	Budget	Mixed	Mixed	Patient
Source	Mixed	Mixed	Government	Mixed	Mixed	Mixed	Government	Mixed	Mixed	Mixed
Status of reform	Phased implementation	Phased implementation	Phased implementation	Phased implementation	Phased implementation	Phased implementation	Full implementation	Phased implementation	Phased implementation	Full implementation
Case-mix classification										
Case-mix in use	Yes	Yes	Yes	Yes	Yes	Yes	Yes	Yes	Yes	Yes
Type of case-mix	AN-DRG	DRG	DRG/HRG	GHM	DRG	DRG	DRG	DRG	DRG	DRG
Quality measure	Quality assurance	Quality assurance	Audit	Clinical evaluation	Audit	Clinical evaluation	Quality assurance	Quality assurance	Clinical evaluation	Peer review organisation

Notes: AN-DRG: Australian national diagnosis-related group.
HRG: Health resource groups.
GHM: *Groupes Homogènes de Maladies.*
DRG: Diagnosis-related group.
Source: Author's evaluations.

by centralised QA (Quality Assurance) programmes by an external agency and enhancement of in-house QA programmes as a condition of funding. Development of a strategy for quality review and assurance should be a priority task under a PPS system" (Scotton and Owens, 1990, Summary Report, p. 47).

A number of states have already advanced to the implementation of a case-mix adjustment in the approach to resource allocation for acute hospital services: in South Australia a proportion of each hospital's budget is determined on the basis of case-mix, and in New South Wales a case-mix adjust-ment factor is integrated into resource allocation for hospital services undertaken at the regional level. In a discussion paper published in March 1993, the Department of Health in Victoria has made a commitment to the introduction of case-mix based budgeting for hospitals from July 1993. In pursuit of the related objectives of improving hospital information and costing systems, together with effectiveness of hospital resource use, the Commonwealth Government has made a further commitment to support the Case-Mix Development Programme for an additional five years.

While most research work to date has been based on HCFA DRGs, a number of recent studies have been specifically targeted on the evaluation of alternative approach to DRG assignment towards the objective of recommending one national standard (Palmer et al., 1990). Based on the findings of these studies, and on input from other relevant groups, the Commonwealth government decided in 1991 to embark on a process of "localising" DRGs in accordance with factors considered to be specific to the Australian hospital environment (McGuire, 1993). The first version of the Australian National DRGs (AN-DRGs) became available in mid-1992.

Belgium

The availability of the appropriate data under the medical registration scheme, together with the positive outcome of a case-mix analysis of activity and costs for Belgian hospitals has facilitated the advancement of proposals to modify the approach to hospital financing (De Moor, 1989; Closon and Roger-France, 1989). A prospective global budget system, which involves differentiation of the budget into separate components for support services and medical services, was introduced in 1982. This financing reform also incorporated the objective of standardizing budgets across hospitals in accor-dance with case-mix and other criteria considered critical to the financing of hospital services. There has been some advancement towards the achievement of this objective with the application of a case-mix adjustment for the budgets for laboratory services in 1990 and radiology services in 1992. Where these services are delivered to in-patients, a case-mix adjusted daily rate for the service now replaces the unadjusted daily rate.

In conjunction with the recommendations for hospital sector reform introduced in 1982, the funda-mental obligation on providers to engage in continual assessment of patterns of clinical service and outcomes was very strongly emphasized. The facility which the DRG system provides for the develop-ment of quality assurance techniques has been recognised as an asset within the Belgian hospital system (Willems, 1989).

United Kingdom

The White Paper "Working for Patients" (1989) presented the blueprint for reform of the National Health Service (NHS) in England and legislation enacted in several stages starting in April 1991 has given effect to the main provisions of these reforms. With regard to the acute hospital sector in particular, the most far-reaching change is the separation of the roles of purchaser and provider of hospital services. There are a number of different ways in which this new type of relationship may be defined, though in each case the hospital fulfils the role of service provider within price and quality controlled service contracts agreed with the purchasing agent. This requires that hospitals define and cost the range of products which they can provide.

Many interesting issues are raised by this latest reform of the NHS in England, some of which are dealt with in an extensive review by the OECD (1992). Of particular interest to the investigation here is the fact that, according to Sanderson (1991), "this new contracting environment has created the potential for a new role for case-mix measures". An interest in this area is not unique to this recent reform as issues concerned with case-mix measurement and application have featured as an integral part of the Department of Health's resource management project since the early 1980s. In the interven-ing decade, extensive research activities have been supported, involving analysis and application of a range of case-mix measures, including DRGs. While the reported evidence "suggests that UK data can be successfully grouped into DRGs and that the resultant groups are medically valid and resource homogeneous", hospitals have complete discretion in the application of case-mix measurement and the case-mix measure of choice (Mills, 1989, p. 10).

Following on the application of the HCFA DRGs within the resource management programme, a series of projects have subsequently been undertaken with the objective of modifying DRGs "to reflect English clinical practice more clearly" (Sanderson, 1991). The results of this investigation were consolidated in 1991 to produce the first version of the Health Resource Groups (HRGs) which are pilot-tested in a number of centres.

Irrespective of the approach adopted to case-mix classification, medical audit is to be a requirement within the NHS. This will involve consultants auditing the process and outcome of the service they provide, and the Royal Colleges being encouraged to make satisfactory audit a precondition for the recognition of clinical training programmes (Schneider et al., 1991).

France

The Programme for Medicalisation of Information Systems (PMSI) has been underway in France since 1982. This programme was among the first European projects to experiment with case-mix measurement and costing within the acute hospital sector. This project was initiated in an era of financing difficulties, and substantial innovations of immediate relevance since that time include a) the implementation of a standardized system for collecting and coding activity data in hospitals (RSS) and b) the implementation of a global budgeting approach for financing public hospitals. Moreover, private hospitals have adopted a case-mix payment since 1992.

With the introduction of budgets for public hospitals in 1984-1985, it was stated government policy to move towards the application of a standardized measure of workload as part of the budgeting process. Advancement towards the achievement of this objective has had to await the enactment of a more recent reform in 1991 which indicated that the process of determining the hospital budget should, in the future, incorporate a discussion of medical activity (Journal officiel, République Française, 2 August 1991). The form that this review of medical activity should take is not specified and will, presumably, be a matter for agreement between the budget negotiators. In 1991, the French Ministry of Health produced an updated version of the case-mix system called Groupes Homogènes de Maladies (GHM). The GHM system is essentially based on the HCFA DRGs, with some local modifications and an integrated mapping facility from local codes to ICD-9-CM.

It is against this background that commentators have noted that "the availability of data on medical information and the utilisation of resources have stimulated the progress of utilisation review" (Boulay, 1988, p. 7). Regardless of the outcome of the choice between different systems, the case-mix approach in France is currently considered to have particularly strong potential in the context of developing techniques for optimising the quality, efficiency and management of hospital service delivery.

Ireland

The approach to financing and funding the health services in Ireland was subjected to examination by the Commission on Health Funding established by the government in 1987. In the report published in 1989, the commission attributed the main weakness in the approach to the funding of hospital services to the fact that "it sustains, over time, the cost differences between efficient hospitals and resource-wasting ones" (Stationery Office, 1989, p. 251). The main recommendation proposed by the commission in response to this problem is summarised as follows:

"Hospitals should receive global budgets for the provision of an agreed service level. The calculation of these budgets should be based on an assessment of the activity level implied by the hospital's agreed role and catchment area, and the case-mix based cost of meeting this" (pp. 257-258).

A DRG-based study of activity and costs in Irish hospitals came to a similar conclusion; it recommended the application of a case-mix adjustment in approaches to resource allocation and management techniques, the combined effect of which would be expected to improve efficiency and facilitate advancement towards the optimisation of care (Wiley and Fetter, 1990). The first step towards "developing a resource allocation system which would link hospital budgets to the type and volume of services to be provided" was taken by the Department of Health in March 1993 with the introduction of a case-mix adjustment for hospital budget (Review Body on Higher Remuneration in the Public Sector, 1990, p. 33).

Since 1990, the Voluntary Health Insurance Board has been using DRGs to analyse claims on a case-mix basis for private hospitals. Case-mix reports are now produced on a quarterly basis and provided to each major private hospital showing ALOS for the top categories of admission, and comparing the results for peer group hospitals on a non-named basis. A case-mix adjustment is also built into payment agreements with a number of major private hospitals to enable adjustments to be made for substantial changes in case-mix intensity over the period of the agreement.

The Irish government attaches high priority to ensuring that an acceptably high standard of care is delivered through the health services. Witness the recent national agreement between all the social partners (government, employers, trade unions, farmers) which included a commitment to the establishment of a Performance Audit Unit within the Department of Health "to assist the Minister in assessing the efficiency and effectiveness of the health services" (Stationery Office, 1991, p. 29).

Norway

For both Norway and Sweden, the starting point for the projects reviewed is a recognition of the need to improve both efficiency and effectiveness within the respective health-care systems. The case-mix measure of choice, the DRG system, is also common to both countries. Beginning in 1991, a pilot exercise has been underway in four hospitals in Norway whereby 40 per cent of the hospital budget is determined on a DRG basis. This pilot project has now been expanded to include eight hospitals. The specific objectives for this initiative have been defined as follows: a) provide an incentive to treat patients with the minimum necessary use of resources; b) utilise the capacity within hospitals to treat more patients; and c) motivate clinicians to use DRGs in monitoring and evaluating their performance on a clinical level (Aas, 1985; Aas et al., 1989; Slattebrekk, 1991). The Norwegian project places particular emphasis on the development of an incentive structure which will promote cost-consciousness in treating patients, and ensure that the most appropriate treatment option is chosen. To assist in the achievement of these objectives, a central peer-review group has been established with a mandate to detect possible poor quality care, and to ensure that hospitals perform in accordance with the intentions of the project (Slattebrekk, 1991).

Sweden

Financing for hospital services in Sweden has been provided on the basis of prospectively determined budgets which include allocations for all expenditure areas, including doctors' fees. With the dawning of the era of cost-containment in the 1980s, the need for tighter control of hospital costs was associated with the introduction of a clinical budgeting approach in some counties. This instrument proved to be somewhat crude, however, for a number of reasons, including the fact the it did not facilitate an accurate estimate of the relationship between inputs used and outputs generated. In addition, the department budgets did not include a cost for the use of internal hospital services which meant that the total cost of service use by the department was underestimated.

It was against this background that the drive for a more fundamental reform of the financing and organisation of the hospital services, in particular, gained momentum towards the end of the 1980s. In recognition of the need for more detailed data about resource use and medical outcome, the study co-ordinated by the Swedish Planning and Rationalisation Institute for Health and Social Services (Spri) set about using DRGs as an analytical tool for generating information combining clinical and resource consumption data (Hakansson, 1988). The structure of hospital service provision in Sweden is currently being re-organised in a number of counties, with the separation of production and financing of services emerging as a key feature of this reorganisation. A review of the reform in Stockholm County Council serves to illustrate the type of approach implemented or being considered in other areas.

Stockholm County Council has made a commitment to the development of an internal market for hospital services within which hospital revenues are to be generated by the sale of services to local health districts. The HCFA DRGs are used as the measure of output on which prices are set prospectively (Hakansson, 1988; Paulson, 1990; Ljunggren and Fries, 1990). In January 1992, when implementation of the new system began, a transitory margin was introduced whereby hospitals would not have to reduce costs by DRG by more than 15 per cent, which means that the fixed DRG prices may not be achieved in all cases. A set of DRG prices has been in use in the clinical departments of general surgery, obstetrics and gynaecology, urology, orthopaedics and cataract surgery in all hospitals throughout the county (OECD, forthcoming). Ambulatory surgery is also covered within the new system with day surgery being reimbursed at 60% of the DRG price fixed for in-patient care. A DRG pricing system has been in operation in all somatic hospitals in Stockholm since January 1993 and it is planned to complete the implementation of the full internal market model by 1995.

With such a major reorganisation of the hospital sector in Sweden, the importance attributed to the tasks of quality assessment and quality assurance has grown considerably (OECD, forthcoming). There have been increasing demands for central follow-up and evaluation which will be concerned with tracing and evaluating the degree of goal achievement, comparing inputs, expenditures and results in different places and for different forms of clinical activity. In particular, the National Board of Health and Welfare and Spri are currently involved in the development of quality indicators which will be used in conjunction with DRG payment in hospitals.

Spain

The 1980s was a period of transition with the beginning of the devolution of responsibility for their respective health care systems to the autonomous regions at the start of the decade, and the extension of compulsory health insurance to the whole population in 1986. Hospitals within the Social Security system are funded on the basis of prospectively determined global budgets for operating costs. Budgets are determined on the basis of historical costs and any savings generated by a hospital must be returned to the central Social Security Fund. When the Social Security system contracts with hospitals outside the system for services, payment is made on the basis of per diem rates which are related to the hospital type.

The fact that the determination of budgets for hospitals in the Social Security system does not take account of activity within the system has been recognised as a problem by the Ministry of Health. This factor, together with the need to improve the efficiency of the health services, increased international experience with case-mix funding models, and the need to use management technology to optimise health-care quality, contributed to the Ministry of Health decision to pursue the development of a new "resource assignment system" for the hospital sector (Esteban, 1992).

In 1991, a project for the development of a "process payment system" was set up with the objective of producing a health product catalogue, based on case-mix measurement, which may serve as a hospital planning, funding and management tool. Thirteen Spanish hospitals are collecting activity and cost data as well as testing analytical tools. HCFA DRGs and Patient Management Categories (PMCs) are being tested as potential measures of case-mix for inclusion in the new system. When the results of these tests are available, the Ministry is expected to draw recommendations on the approach to case-mix measurement and system design which will enable the development of a process payment approach for implementation in acute hospitals.

Catalonia was the first autonomous region with responsibility for health care. In a period of expenditure restraint in the mid-1980s, the objectives of improving hospital management and identifying solutions to recognised areas of inefficiency became a priority (Casas, 1989; 1991). It was in this context that the application of case-mix-based approaches to resource management came to be developed and tested. The HCFA DRGs have been used in Barcelona since the mid-1980s and this initiative has now advanced to the development of allocation models for the evaluation of relative efficiency and budget allocation between hospitals (Ibern *et al.*, 1991). In pursuing the development of these applications, the introduction of utilisation review programmes and training programmes for managers and clinicians has been recognised as critical to ensure appropriate use of the information being produced and the techniques developed (Casas, 1989).

Portugal

Hospital services are funded on the basis of prospectively determined global budgets which are allocated to hospitals on an annual basis. In 1981 the Ministry of Health made a commitment to the principle of output-based funding for hospital care within the constraint of overall budget neutrality. Following an extensive research and development programme involving the development of hospital information systems, the updating of coding systems and the introduction of training and education programmes, a resource allocation model within which a designated proportion of the hospital budget is estimated on a DRG basis was put in place in 1990.

The model applied may be summarised as follows:

"Appropriations for each hospital for inpatient care under the National Health Service are determined by multiplying its expected number of cases times its case-mix index and times its base-rate which is partly related to the hospital's specific costs. Adjustments to the budget allocations are applied to account for outlier and transfer cases and to ensure overall neutrality of the NHS budget" (Bentes and Gonsalves, 1992).

This output-based resource allocation model for acute hospital services will continue to be developed in line with on-going assessments of the effectiveness of the system which has been put in place. While ambulatory services continue to be funded from the national budget on the basis of historic expenditure adjusted for inflation, the inclusion of this sector within a comprehensive output-based funding model is recognised as an important objective for future development.

One response to the recognition that quality of care must be protected and enhanced under the new funding system is evident in the current application of a system of utilisation review. The fact that morbidity coding is done by doctors in Portuguese hospitals would be expected to add a very valuable perspective to this process, particularly on such issues as data coverage and data quality. The long-term goals for system development are also concerned with facilitating a relationship between the regional resource allocation system and case level quality assessment and utilisation review (Vertrees and Manton, 1991).

There is some evidence, therefore, that all of the countries listed in Table 2 are working towards combining case-mix measurement and quality assurance/assessment procedures in the interests of improving the efficiency of their respective approaches to financing hospital care. Several countries have, however, concentrated attention on the potential for application of case-mix measures for achieving improvements in approaches to planning and internal hospital management. These objectives are not in any way mutually exclusive, and many researchers have investigated approaches to the achievement of both goals. The conclusion of this review will be limited to this subset of countries which includes Finland, Italy, the Netherlands and Switzerland.

Finland

The drive for cost-containment at the hospital and inter-hospital level has focused attention on the need to improve the efficiency of internal hospital departments. This has stimulated the development of a case-mix application for management techniques within Finnish hospitals (Brommels, 1988). In 1990 a new Hospital Act was enacted with the objective of changing the structure of financing of public hospitals to ensure that the revenue budget was more closely related to productivity and efficiency standards. This reform, together with the new State Subsidy Act which started in 1993, is now focusing attention on the potential which may be offered by a case-mix classification scheme like the DRGs for the required product descriptions of hospital services (Brommels, 1990; OECD, forthcoming).

Italy

The recognition that comparisons at the specialty or hospital level must control for the heterogeneity of patients treated, was the starting point for a number of important studies of hospital case-mix (Taroni, 1990). The research conducted by Taroni and his colleagues concentrated on examining the potential of measures like the DRGs and/or Disease Staging for estimating the relationship between resource use variables and key independent variables so that some support might be given to management within the hospital in correcting for observed deficiencies in performance. The importance of combining good management with quality care is consistently emphasized in this research. Taroni (1990) recommends that "selection of the few 'relevant' DRGs which account for a significant amount of resources, will provide 'good' DRGs for evaluation research, showing clear-cut definitions of the range of acceptable variation in the care process, more homogeneity of the patient clinical characteristics and low 'provider uncertainty', thus allowing for firm and valid criteria for process evaluation" (p. 64).

The Netherlands

While according priority to the development of effective tools for management support, including utilisation review and quality assurance, the research emanating from the Netherlands has consistently emphasized the importance of flexibility in any patient classification systems (PCSs) used (van Dijk and Voss, 1990). Experimentation with the DRG system has proceeded in association with the development of local schemes. Dutch hospital managers are fortunate in having access to relatively comprehensive data bases on activity and service use within the hospital. A critical issue for the future, however, will be the development of appropriate patient classification models to enable the available information to be consolidated and made accessible to managers within a meaningful and intelligible framework.

A detailed study of the potential for case-mix measurement and application in Switzerland, using DRGs, was published by Paccaud and Schenker in 1989. This extensive analysis of hospital activity explains the integrity of this case-mix application within the Swiss health system. A core conclusion and recommendation arising from this study is summarised by Schenker (1991) as follows:

"The use of groups of patients as budgetary unit for management and as indicator for the allocation of resources within the hospital grid network, appears possible. Also the DRGs, or a regrouping based on these, appear entirely appropriate to the planning of beds or of hospitals, as well as to studies evaluating their performances" (p. 3).

Discussion

The OECD countries included in this review have different types of health-care systems. While different systems may share elements of particular health system models, national characteristics and culture demand that the precise specification of any model within a national framework must be specific to that context.

Given this starting point, therefore, what is quite surprising is the high degree of commonalty in evidence for the programmes or proposals examined. With specific reference to the hospital services, whether the focus is on financing or management, all countries share a common quest for improvements in both the efficiency and effectiveness of performance. While the specific avenues under consideration for the achievement of these goals may vary, there is general recognition that an appropriate measure of case-mix may provide a useful tool. The case-mix measure of choice is not as important to this investigation as is the generalised recognition of the potential power of the technique when part of a comprehensive approach to management or financing reform.

While recognising the importance of ensuring that appropriate quality assurance measures form an integral part of any reforms undertaken, there is some disparity in the systems reviewed with regard to the approach to quality of care assessment under consideration. A number of countries, Portugal and England for example, have implemented programmes on utilisation review and audit, respectively. Proposals emanating from other countries have not progressed beyond the recognition that quality assurance is a desirable component of programme reform. This vagueness does not in any way represent a lack of commitment, but may be more a function of the absence of data needed to pursue this objective.

The experiences presented above suggest that while countries may vary in the type of health system supported and the objectives for change, they may share common approaches to the development and application of measures of hospital case-mix. From this background we are encouraged to ask whether countries might also, in time, come to share similar approaches to quality assurance in the context of diversity. If this works for techniques like case-mix measurement, then there is every reason to believe that it could also work for quality assurance measures. Theoretical and operational issues arising with the measurement of quality have been addressed by researchers and academics for a long time. The question of application has now become more widespread with the generalised acceptance of the principle that quality must be protected and enhanced, and that programmes of reform should include an explicit quality of care component.

The United States is still the only country to have evaluated, with positive results, a case-mix based PPS which was implemented in conjunction with a programme of quality assurance. The experience of quality assurance programmes may not be very extensive, but is expanding at a very rapid pace in other countries as well. Further investigation in this area might therefore be well rewarded by specific concentration on the tools of quality assurance and their potential for application in different types of health-care systems across national boundaries.

Conclusions and recommendations

In conclusion, two questions may be presented. First, is it safe today to assume that quality – in every meaning and connotation of the word – has a permanent and prominent place on national health-care agendas? And second, have we finally succeeded in refuting the assumption that quality inevitably strains the budget?

Evidence suggests that these battles have essentially been won. What is particularly exciting about many recent reforms in hospitals is the fact that researchers and policy-makers have come to the same conclusion: quality is not an optional extra; it is an essential ingredient of any reform agenda.

Cost-containment and control sat at the top of national health-care agendas since the 1970s. Indeed the legacy of the past two decades risked a devaluation of quality as an essential part of the health-care system. The debate would now, however, seem to have matured with experience and moved beyond the simplistic level to a degree of sophistication more appropriate to the complexity of the issues involved. The cautionary warning sounded by Vertrees (Vertrees and Manton, 1991) that "incentives to use resources efficiently are simultaneously incentives to under-provide services" has been clearly noted (p. 16). There is now ample evidence to suggest that the twin objectives of efficiency and effectiveness have moved to the top of the agenda, bringing with them an unavoidable concern with the quantification and evaluation of the outputs and the outcomes of the health-care system (Wiley, 1992). The fact that a framework for measuring outputs must be put in place if outcomes are to be accurately assessed has ensured that measures of case-mix and quality are complementary components of a comprehensive health-care policy.

The challenge which now emerges is to facilitate movement from the *why* to the *how* of quality assurance. Towards this end, Schneider *et al.* (1991) recommend that:

"The guidelines for European health service treatment baskets therefore should also contain rules for quality assurance. International quality indicators, exchange programmes for doctors and nurses between hospitals of different countries, international vocational programmes, and research programmes might help to develop quality standards for facilities, manpower, medical equipment, and serving process" (p. 99).

The pursuit of this objective leads, inevitably, to the call for better information on tools and techniques, together with a pooling of results to facilitate speedier advancement. A review of this nature has been limited by the scarcity of such data at the international level. As the level of expertise and application develops, available data sources are likely to expand accordingly.

Those interested in embarking upon this mission, however, may be chastened by the comment that:

"The assessment of outcome is too important to be left to clinicians, and certainly too subtle to be left to health economists, administrators and epidemiologists (...). It cannot be left to any one group because it affects us all – politicians, professionals and the public" (Clare, 1990, p. 109).

Given a literal interpretation of this statement, the research community might be forgiven for giving up before beginning. The so-called rebirth of interest in this objective, which has accompanied many of the recent reforms taking place in health services across the OECD, demands, however, that serious attempts be made towards its achievement.

Acknowledgements

The support and assistance of the following colleagues is gratefully acknowledged: J.-P. Poullier (OECD), M. Bentes (Portugal), M. Casas and P. Ibern (Spain), P. Devereux (Ireland), S. Hakansson (Sweden), J. Hofdijk (Netherlands), L. Jenkins and H. Sanderson (England), G. Neubauer (Germany), J-M Rodrigues (France), O. Slattebrekk (Norway). Any outstanding errors of commission and/or ommission remain the responsibility of the author.

Bibliography

Aas, I.H.M. (1985), *DRG: Diagnose Relaterte Grupper – En Litteraturoversikt,* Report, 3/85, Norsk Institutt for Sykehusforskning, Oslo.

Aas, I.H.M., Freeman, J.L., Palmer, G.R. and Fetter, R.B. (1989), *The Making of Norwegian DRGs,* Report 3/89, Norwegian Institute for Hospital Research, Oslo.

Bentes, M. and Gonsalves, M. da Luz (1992), "DRG-Based Funding in Portugal: Two Years After", Proceeding of the Third EURODRG Workshop: Case-Mix Management in Europe, Madrid, 21-22 May.

Bentes, M., Urbano, J., Do Carmo Carvalho, M. and Tranquada, S. (1991), "Using DRGs to Fund Hospitals in Portugal: An Evaluation of the Experience", paper prepared for the Second EURODRG Workshop, Dublin, April. *Diagnosis-Related Groups in Europe, Uses and Perspectives,* M. Casas and M.M. Wiley (dir. publ.)

Bentes, M., Urbano, J. and Hindle, D. (1989), "Output-Based Funding in Portugal: Taking the First Steps", in *The Management and Financing of Hospital Services,* Conference Proceedings, Washington.

Boulay, F. (1988), "DRGs, Information System and Utilization Review in French Hospitals", in *The Management and Financing of Hospital Services,* Conference Proceedings, Sydney, 18-20 February.

Brommels, M. (1988), "Towards Patient Orientated Hospital Management; Purpose, Organization and Early Results of the Finnish DRG Project", in *The Management and Financing of Hospital Services,* Conference Proceedings, Sydney, 18-20 February.

Brommels, M. (1990), "The Blue White Paper. Case Remixing in Finnish Health Care", Proceedings of *The 6th International Working Conference,* Patient Classification Systems – Europe, Saint-Etienne, France, September.

Brook, R. (1987), "Case-Mix Measurement and Quality of Care Symposium", *Health Care Financing Review,* Annual Supplement.

Casas, M. (1989), "Application of DRGs in Hospital Management in Spain", in *The Third International Conference on the Management and Financing of Hospital Services,* Conference Proceedings, Washington.

Casas, M. (1991), *Los Grupos Relacionados con el Diagnostico, Experiencia y Perspectivas de Utilizacion,* Masson, Barcelona.

Clare, A. W. (1990), "Some Conclusions", in Hopkins, A. and Costain D. (eds.), *Measuring the Outcomes of Medical Care,* The Royal College of Physicians of London.

Closon, M.C. and Roger-France, F.H. (1989), "Structures des pathologies et financement des soins de santé", in F.H. Roger-France, G. De Moor, J. Hofdijk, L. Jenkins (eds), *Diagnosis Related Groups in Europe,* 2nd edition.

Codman, E.A. (1914), "The Product of a Hospital", *Surgery, Gynaecology and Obstetrics,* 18 (January-June): 491-96.

Codman, E.A. (1916), *A Study in Hospital Efficiency. The First Five Years,* Thomas Todd, Boston.

Coulam, R.F. and Gaumer, G.L. (1992), "Medicare's prospective payment system: A critical appraisal", *Health Care Financing Review 1991,* Annual Supplement: 45-77. HCFA Pub. No. 03322. Office of Research and Demonstrations, Health Care Financing Administration, Washington, US Government Printing Office, March.

De Moor, G. (1989), "Observations on reliability in the registration of diagnoses and operating loan procedures in Belgium", in F.H. Roger-France, G. De Moor, J. Hofdijk, L. Jenkins (eds), *Diagnosis Related Groups in Europe,* 2nd edition.

Donabedian, A. (1966), "Evaluating the Quality of Medical Care", *Milibank Memorial Fund Quarterly,* 44 (3, Part 2): 166-206, July.

Donabedian, A. (1987), "Commentary on Some Studies of the Quality of Care", *Health Care Financing Review,* Annual Supplement.

Duckett, S.J. (1988), "DRGs in Victoria", in *The Management and Financing of Hospital Services,* Conference Proceedings, Sydney, 18-20 February.

Esteban Garcia, J. (1992), "Application of a Process Payment System in National (SNS) Hospitals", EC Concerted Action: Use of DRGs to Support Hospital Sector Management in the European Community, Third EURODRG Workshop, Madrid.

Fetter, R.B., Shin, Y., Freeman, J.L., Averill, R.F. and Thomson, J.D. (1980), "Case Mix Definition By Diagnosis Related Groups", *Medical Care,* 18, 2 (Supplement), December: 1-53.

Fetter, R.B., J.D. Thompson and R.F. Averill (1981), *Development, Testing, and Evaluation of a Prospective Case-Payment Reimbursement System,* Final Report, Health Care Financing Administration, Department of Health and Human Services.

Hakansson, S. (1988), "DRGs in Sweden – Update", in *The Management and Financing of Hospital Services,* Conference Proceedings, Sydney, 18-20 February.

Health Care Financing Administration, Report to Congress (1991), *Impact of the Medicare Hospital Prospective Payment System,* Annual Report, Washington, D.C.

HMSO (1989), *Working for Patients,* London, Her Majesty's Stationery Office.

Hornbrook, M.C. (1985), "Techniques for Assessing Hospital Case Mix", *Ann. Rev. Public Health,* 6:295-324.

Hornbrook, M.C. and Goldfarb M.G. (1981), "Patterns of Obstetrical Care in Hospitals", *Medical Care,* 19, p. 55.

Ibern, P., Bisbel J. and Casas, M. (1991), "The Development of cost information by DRG - Experience in a Barcelona hospital", *Health Policy,* Vol. 17(2), pp. 179-194.

Kahn, K.L., Rubenstein, L.V., Draper, D., Kosecoff, J., Rogers, W.H., Keeler, E.B. and Brook, R.H. (1990*a*), "The Effects of the DRG-Based Prospective Payment System on Quality of Care for Hospitalized Medicare Patients. An Introduction to the Series", *Journal of the American Medical Association,* October 17, 264: 1953-1955.

Kahn, K.L., Keeler, E.B., Sherwood, M.J., Rogers, W.H., Draper, D., Bentow, S.S., Reinish, E.J., Rubenstein, L.V., Kosecoff, J. and Brook, R.H. (1990*b*), "Comparing Outcomes of Care Before and After Implementation of the DRG-Based Prospective Payment System", *Journal of the American Medical Association,* October 17, 264: 1984-1988.

Kahn, K.L., Rogers, W.H., Rubenstein, L.V., Sherwood, M.J., Reinisch, E.J., Keeler, E.B., Draper, D., Kosecoff, J. and Brook, R.H. (1990*c*), "Measuring Quality of Care With Explicit Process Criteria Before and After Implementation of the DRG-Based Prospective Payment System", *Journal of the American Medical Association,* October 17, 264: 1969-1973.

Keeler, E.B., Kahn, K.L., Draper, D., Sherwood, M.J., Rubenstein, L.V., Reinisch, E.J., Kosecoff, J. and Brook, R.H. (1990), "Changes in Sickness at Admission Following the Introduction of the Prospective Payment System", *Journal of the American Medical Association,* October 17, 264: 1962-1968,.

Kosecoff, J., Kahn, K.L., Rogers, W.H., Reinisch, E.J., Sherwood, M.J., Rubenstein, L.V., Draper, D., Roth, C.P., Chew, C. and Brook, R.H. (1990), "Prospective Payment System and Impairment at Discharge", *Journal of the American Medical Association,* October 17, 264: 1980-1983.

Krakauer, R. (1987), "Case-Mix Measurement and Quality of Care Symposium", *Health Care Financing Review,* Annual Supplement.

Lave, J.R. and Leinhardt, S. (1976), "The Cost and Length of a Hospital Stay", *Inquiry,* 13, p. 327.

Ljunggren, G. and Fries B.E. (1990), "International Validation of RUGs in Long-Term Care", paper presented at *The 6th International Working Conference, Patient Classification Systems Europe,* Saint-Etienne, France, 26-29 September.

Luke, R.D. (1979), "Dimensions in Hospital Care Mix Measurement", *Inquiry,* 16, p. 38.

McGuire, T.E. (1993), "DRG Evolution", in Casas, M. and Wiley, M.M. (ed.), *Diagnosis Related Groups in Europe: Uses and Perspectives,* Madrid.

Mills, I. (1989), *Past Progress and Future Plans, A Mid-Term Report from the Director of Resource Management,* London, NHS Management Executive, HMSO.

Neubauer, G. (1991), "Patient Management Categories in Germany", paper prepared for the 2nd EURODRG Workshop, Dublin, April.

OECD (1985), *Measuring Health Care 1960-1983 Expenditure: Costs and Performance,* Paris.

OECD (1992), *The Reform of Health Care: A Comparative Analysis of Seven Countries,* Paris.

OECD (1993), *OECD Health Systems: Facts and Trends 1960-1991,* Paris (2 vol.)

OECD (forthcoming), *The Reform of Health Care – A Review of 17 OECD Countries,* Paris.

Paccaud, F. and Schenker, L. (1989), *DRG: Perspectives d'utilisation,* Institut suisse de la santé publique et des hôpitaux.

Palmer, G.R. (1990), "The Funding of Hospitals Using Diagnosis Related Groups: Problems and Solutions", in Selby-Smith, C. (ed), *Economics and Health 1989,* Proceedings of the Eleventh Australian Conference of Health Economists, PSMI, Monash University, Melbourne.

Palmer, G., Reid, B. and Aisbett, C. (1990), *The Refinement and Adaptation of Diagnosis Related Groups for Use in Australia,* Interim Report to the Commonwealth Department of Community Services and Health and to the Australian Grouper Consensus Conference, the University of New South Wales, Canberra.

Paulson, E.M. (1990), *DRGs in Sweden – Adaptation and Applications on Patient Discharge Data,* The Swedish Planning and Rationalization Institute for the Health and Social Services, Stockholm.

Programme for Economic and Social Progress (1991), Stationery Office, Dublin.

ProPAC (Prospective Payment Assessment Commission) (1988), *Report and Recommendations to the Secretary,* US Department of Health and Human Services, March.

ProPAC (1990), *Medicare Prospective Payment and the American Health Care System,* Report to the Congress, June.

ProPAC (1991*a*), *Report and Recommendations to the Congress,* March.

ProPAC (1991*b*), *Medicare and the American Health Care System,* Report to the Congress, June.

République Française : Loi N° 91-748 du 31 juillet 1991, portant sur la réforme hospitalière; Loi N° 91-738 du 31 juillet 1991, portant sur diverses mesures d'ordre social.

Rogers, W.H., Draper, D., Kahn, K.L., Keeler, E.B., Rubenstein, L.V., Kosecoff, J. and Brook, R.H. (1990), "Quality of Care before and after Implementation of the DRG-Based Prospective Payment System, a Summary of Effects", *Journal of the American Medical Association,* October 17, 264: 1989-1994.

Rubenstein, L.V., Kahn, K.L., Reinisch, E.J., Sherwood, M.J., Rogers, W.H., Kamberg, C., Draper, D. and Brook, R.H. (1990), "Changes in Quality of Care for Five Diseases Measured by Implicit Review 1981 to 1986", *Journal of the American Medical association,* October 17, 264: 1974-1979.

Russell, L.B. (1989), *Medicare's New Prospective Payment System: Is it Working?,* The Brookings Institution, Washington, D.C.

Sanderson, H.F. (1991), "The UK Approach to Costing by DRG", Journée PCS-DRG: Des outils pour faire quoi?, Lausanne.

Schenker, L. (1991), "Perspectives d'utilisation des DRG dans le Canton de Vaud", *DRG News,* No. 2, January.

Schneider, M., Dennerlein, R.K.H., Kose, A. and Scholtes, L. (1991), *Health Care "Baskets",* Study for the Commission of the European Community, Augsburg.

Scotton, R.B. and Owens, H.J. (1990), *Case Payment in Australian Hospitals: Issues and Options,* report of a Study Funded by the Commonwealth Department of Community Services and Health.

Slattebrekk, O.V. (1991), "Introducing Financial Incentives in Hospitals – Prospective Payment by DRG in Norway", paper prepared for the *2nd EURODRG Workshop,* Dublin, April.

Stationery Office (1989), *Report of the Commission on Health Funding,* Dublin,.

Stationery Office (1990), *Review Body on Higher Remuneration in the Public Sector,* Report No. 32, Hospital Consultants, Dublin.

Stationery Office (1991), *Programme for Economic and Social Progress,* Dublin.

Taroni, F. (1990), "Using Diagnosis-Related Groups for Performance Evaluation of hospital care", in Leidl, R., Potthoff, C. and Schwefel, D. (eds.), *European Approaches to Patient Classification Systems,* Springer-Verlag.

van Dijk, P. and Voss, G. (1990), "Experiences with the Introduction of DRGs in the Maastricht University Hospital", Proceedings of *The 6th international Working Conference,* Patient Classification Systems – Europe, Saint-Etienne, France.

Vertrees, J.C. and Manton, K.G. (1991), "Using Case-Mix for Resource Allocation", paper prepared for the *2nd EURODRG Workshop,* Dublin, April.

Vuori, H. and Roger, F. (1989), "Issues in Quality Assurance – The European Scene", *Quality Assurance in Health Care,* Vol. 1, No. 2/3, pp. 125-135.

Wilensky, G.R. (1990), "Medicare at 25. Better Value and Better Care", *Journal of the American Medical Association,* October 17, 264:1995.6-1997.

Wiley, M.M. (1990), "Patient Classification Systems: Overview of Experiments and Applications in Europe", in Leidl, R., Potthoff, C. and Schwefel, D. (eds.), *European Approaches to Patient Classification Systems,* Springer-Verlag.

Wiley, M.M. (1992), "Hospital Financing Reform and Case-Mix Measurement: An International Review", *Health Care Financing Review,* Summer.

Wiley, M.M. and Fetter, R.B. (1990), *Measuring Activity and Costs in Irish Hospitals: A Study of Hospital Case Mix,* The Economic and Social Research Institute, Dublin.

Wiley, M.M. and Leidl, R. (1989), "Performance Measurement in Hospitals: The Application of Diagnosis Related Groups", in Leidl, R., John, J. and Schwefel, D. (eds.), *Performance Indicators in Health Care: Selected Readings on Concepts and Applications,* MEDIS-GSF, Munich.

Willems, J.L. (1989), "Use of Diagnosis Related Groups for Internal Hospital Management", in Roger-France, F.H., De Moor, G., Hofdijk, J. and Jenkins L. (eds), *Diagnosis Related Groups in Europe,* 2nd edition.

HEALTH MAINTENANCE ORGANIZATIONS:
IS THE UNITED STATES EXPERIENCE APPLICABLE ELSEWHERE?

by

Harold S. Luft

The rapidly rising cost of medical care has become a major issue for many developed nations. In recent years, the United States, which spends a comparatively large percentage of its GNP on care, has thus been led to place particular emphasis on the issue of cost-containment. A wide range of containment policies have been and are being tried at federal, state and private level – with varying results. Increased attention to competitive forces in the 1980s has replaced the direct regulatory efforts of the 1970s. Major features of the increasingly competitive environment are the newer forms of payment systems, such as preferred provider organisations (PPOs), managed care plans and, most notably, health maintenance organisations (HMOs) which have a long history of serving a relatively small segment of the population. There is substantial evidence that some HMOs provide comprehensive medical care for their enrollees at lower cost than do fee-for-service providers. Further, HMOs are seen as being instrumental in increasing competitive pressures on conventional providers. Finally, while there is much discussion of these newer systems, there is little solid research on their performance; for this reason, HMOs have been singled out as the main focus of what follows.

As the costs of care increases in developed nations, international interest in HMOs rises accordingly. This article will first briefly summarise the existing evidence on HMO performance in the United States – with the proviso that it must be viewed in the context of the changing US medical care system. It is an open question, moreover, whether past performances of HMOs are useful for predicting their future – even in the United States. By way of conclusion, those issues which must be considered if the US HMO model were to be transferred to other nations will be outlined.

Existing evidence on HMO performance

HMOs are often discussed as if they were simple, homogeneous organisations, easily replicated, and well understood. In reality, each HMO is a highly complex combination of economic incentives, bureaucratic structures and personalities. Many varieties of HMOs exist and even similarly structured plans perform differently (much as do similarly structured industrial firms), their performance depending in part on the local environment. In short, we know relatively little about exactly how they work. To interpret for policy purposes the research on HMOs, one must generalise from a relatively small number of carefully studied cases keeping in mind the inherent limitations of such an approach when developing policy options.

A generic definition of HMOs

HMOs are specifically defined for the purposes of federal and state regulatory agencies, but a generic definition of an HMO includes the following characteristics:

- The HMO assumes a contractual responsibility to provide or ensure the delivery of a stated range of health services, including at least physician and hospital care.
- The HMO serves a defined group of voluntarily enrolled subscribers.

- The HMO requires a fixed, periodic payment to the organisation that is independent of the use of services. There may be small charges related to utilisation, but these are relatively insignificant.
- The HMO assumes at least part of the financial risk and/or gain in the provision of services.

Contractual responsibility implies that the HMO enrollee has a legal right to medical care provided by the HMO. By contrast, in the usual situation, the medical care provider has the right to accept the patient but is under no legal obligation, except in emergencies, to provide care. Someone enrolled in a conventional health insurance plan has the right to be reimbursed for the cost of services, but it is the consumer's responsibility to find a provider. The existence of an enrolled, defined population means that the HMO knows its obligations in advance, and can estimate the probable demand for its services. Voluntary enrolment implies that the consumer can periodically choose between the HMO and a conventional fee-for-service reimbursement plan. It also includes situations in which people may be forced to be in an HMO, but have a choice among several HMOs. The definition is intended to exclude mandatory enrolment in systems without alternatives, such as the military and student health clinics. The fixed, periodic payment, or capitation (independent of the quantity of services provided), implies that for a given enrollee, the HMO does not gain any substantial revenue by providing more services. In the long run, however, an HMO may gain enrollees by offering more services, and it will lose members if it noticeably underserves them. Finally, financial risk implies that the HMO will suffer or benefit financially from its decisions to provide services and attract enrollees.

This definition purposely allows for considerable variation in the organisational characteristics of the HMO. For example, physicians could practice together in a clinic setting, either as employees of the HMO or as a legally distinct medical group contracting with the HMO. The first form is often termed a "staff model" and the second a "group model" plan. Both varieties are sometimes lumped together under the label "prepaid group practice" or PGP. Alternatively, the HMO could contract with physicians who also maintain substantial fee-for-service (FFS) practices, often called an "individual practice association", or IPA. In some cases, IPAs contract primarily with FFS-oriented groups of physicians, and this is often termed a "network model", because of its network of independent clinics.

The evidence of HMO performance in several different dimensions is discussed in varying degrees of detail in several publications (Luft, 1980a, 1981, 1987; Wolinsky, 1980; Morrison and Luft, 1990; Burns and Wholey, 1991). This article will briefly focus on utilisation, quality of care, socio-demographic differences, consumer satisfaction, trends in costs, and competitive effects. In general, the discussion has been limited to published research studies with appropriate analytical methods and controls. This implies that at time, only a handful of studies are available, covering only a limited number of HMOs.

Cost differences

Available evidence is generally quite convincing: the total medical care costs of HMO enrollees is lower than that of fee-for-services users covered by conventional reimbursement insurance. These lower costs persist even after adjusting for differences in age and sex across enrollee groups. The voluntary enrolment aspect of HMOs may naturally lead to selection bias in which the risk of requiring medical care is not equal across plans. In some instances HMOs attract healthier enrollees. The substantial policy issues raised by selection bias will be explored below (see Wilensky and Rossiter, 1983; Hellinger, 1987). Enrollees in PGPs consistently have total medical care costs 10-40% lower than do people who receive care in FFS plans. These cost figures include premiums, out-of-pocket costs for copayments, and the cost of services not provided by the plan. The evidence for lower costs among enrollees in IPAs is less clear, largely because of greater variability among IPAs. While most of these studies observed people choosing various plans, one, very large, carefully done study by the Rand Corporation involved the random assignment of people to an HMO or to conventional insurance plans with FFS providers, in which HMO costs were in the order to 25% lower than with extensive FFS coverage (Manning et al., 1984).

Types of medical care utilisation

The lower overall costs for HMO enrollees seem to be primarily attributable to lower rates of hospital use; the number of ambulatory care visits per enrollee do not show consistent differences by delivery system. HMO physicians seem less inclined to hospitalise their patients, but once admitted,

HMO-enrollee hospital stays are not shown to be shorter. Unfortunately, the different hospital admission rates result in case-mix differences, so aggregate measures of length of stay are misleading. With a few notable exceptions, HMOs do not own their hospitals, so cost differences cannot be attributed to more efficient methods of delivering a day of hospital care. The Kaiser Permanente plans in California (belonging to a large, mature HMO which owns 18 hospitals), regionalise their services and provide less duplication of specialised equipment, such as CT scanners and open heart surgery units, than does the "system" of community hospitals (Luft and Crane, 1980). There is also little evidence that physicians practising as a group realise economies-of-scale in the production of office visits relative to practitioners in separate offices; the PGP savings seem to be associated with greater control over the use of services.

Quality

The technical quality of care in HMOs (in contrast to the patient's perception of care, to be discussed below) is generally comparable to that delivered in FFS settings. (See the above reviews and Cunningham and Williamson, 1980.) This seems to be the case whether one uses measures of process (such as whether the appropriate tests were ordered), or of outcomes, (such as mortality or morbidity). The aforementioned Rand study has the most detailed measures of health status-at-enrolment and outcome measures of health after 3-5 years in the experiment (Ware *et al.*, 1986, report the outcome results of the study). In general, health status was comparable for enrollees in the HMO and FFS plans, even though HMO enrollees utilised fewer services. An exception: low-income enrollees who were in poor health at the beginning of the experiment did less well in the HMO than in the FFS plan.

Socio-economic differences

This finding, that poor enrollees who were initially sick had worse outcomes in HMOs, raises the question of how well HMOs serve the poor. Most HMOs were developed for employee groups, usually blue-collar workers, but some plans enrol substantial numbers of white-collar and professional workers. In general, however, upper-income people find the restrictions imposed by the HMO style of practice less convenient, while the cost savings are not as important to them. Moreover, most HMOs have not positioned themselves to serve those too poor to pay the necessary premiums, typically those who work for employers unwilling to provide insurance coverage. In some states, the state Medicaid programme for the poor has enrolled individuals in HMOs under special contracts. Sometimes these contracts include provision for special outreach services and other benefits not provided to the average employed enrollee. (In fact the plan studied by the Rand group had such a contract with the Medicaid programme in the state of Washington, but the experimental enrollees were not eligible for such special services which might have made a difference in their ability to gain access to the plan's providers.) Some state contracts with HMOs have been long-standing, with quite good results, but in a few instances there have been major problems, generally due to the structure of the state plan, rather than to the HMOs *per se*.

Consumer satisfaction

Consumer satisfaction is a crucial measure of HMO performance. PGPs tend to score worse than FFS providers in various aspects of satisfaction, such as time between calling and scheduling an appointment, physician-patient interaction, information transfer, and perceived quality of care. On the other hand, PGPs score better with respect to doctor punctuality and financial coverage. One way of aggregating these divergent perspectives is by examining how people "vote with their feet". In general, HMOs have increased their share of enrollees within employee groups that are offered a choice. It appears that the lower enrollee cost outweighs the other disadvantages for many potential enrollees.

Trends in costs

The lower cost for HMO enrollees is only one aspect of the cost question, the rate of increase is also important. There is no evidence that HMO costs have increased more slowly than costs in the FFS sector (Luft, 1980a; Newhouse et al., 1985). However, even if the rate of growth is the same, 20% lower costs year after year are not insignificant. The comparable trends in premiums may hide truly divergent patterns in costs; over time, HMOs have tended to expand coverages and benefits while FFS plans have introduced restrictions. Furthermore, the comparable rate of growth in HMO costs could be attributed to several factors that may be changing. In most parts of the United States, there has been relatively little competition among HMOs so a plan could merely let its premiums rise along with FFS premiums. In addition, the growth of medical technology is partially responsible for cost increases. The HMO market share (under 15%) has been too small to influence product development, but with the advent of prospective payment, there are much stronger incentives for manufacturers to design effi-ciency-enhancing innovations rather than just quality-enhancing ones; HMOs may be more inclined to adopt those likely to reduce total costs, rather than just cost per admission.

Competitive effects

Finally, it has often been suggested that the development and growth of HMOs would lead conventional FFS providers and insurers to adopt more cost-containing strategies to maintain their competitive position. In fact, the available evidence from the late 1970s and early 1980s suggests no such competitive effect, or even its opposite – increased cost and hospital use. As providers sought to make up for revenue lost to HMOs, they increased prices more rapidly and provided even more services per capita in the remaining FFS population (Luft, Maerki, Trauner, 1986; McLaughlin et al., 1984). It is clear from observing the present scene, however, that the growth of HMOs has engendered an increased competitive process. Both HMOs and FFS providers and insurers now place much greater emphasis on marketing. An increased emphasis on cost-containment by employers may ultimately restructure the medical care environment so that HMO competition will lead to lower community-wide costs. To understand these changes, however, one must consider the changing health care environ-ment in the United States.

The past and present medical care systems in the United States

One must take into account changes in the overall health care system, payment incentives, and regulation in the United States as we review available evidence on HMO performance. In contrast to current news clippings and anecdotal stories, much of the research on HMOs used data from the years before the implementation of the federal prospective payment programme for Medicare patients (pre 1984); it has generally focused on what might be called first and second generation HMOs. These are plans that were developed before the 1970s when the growth of federal interest in HMOs led to grant and loan programmes encouraging HMO development followed by the elimination of such support in the 1980s. Thus, the research is based upon a subset of HMOs situated in a health care financing and marketing era that no longer exists. This section will first outline the earlier environment and characteris-tics of the typical "mature" HMO serving as the basis for most of the analytic studies. Next, it will discuss some of the current changes in the medical care market, the new HMOs entering the market, and some of the potential implications of the new situation.

Medical Care Financing in the United States up to the Early 1980s

Medical care in the United States is primarily financed through four major "systems": a) Medicare, a federal programme for almost all the elderly and permanently disabled; b) Medicaid, a federal-state programme for the poor; c) private insurance, usually subsidised in part by employers; d) public health clinics and hospitals, for those without other coverage. With some exceptions, the public system of hospitals and clinics is concentrated in major urban areas and is relatively unconnected from the other systems, all of which, to some extent, share the same providers. That is, a physician would be likely to treat patients with Medicare, Medicaid, and private insurance, admitting them to a community hospital, but the same physician would probably not see patients in a public clinic or county hospital. Until the early 1980s, Medicare, Medicaid, and most private insurance essentially paid provider and hospital bills (*i.e.* charges) or reimbursed them for costs according to certain formulas. This general payment system is often referred to as cost-based reimbursement. Under this system, there was little incentive for providers to develop more efficient methods of production because any savings would soon be recaptured by the reimbursing agency. Increased legitimate costs (*i.e.* within the appropriate categories) would always be paid by reimbursement. More important, there were no incentives under either cost- or charge-based systems to reduce the use of medical care services. Instead, to the extent that a patient was fully insured, a physician could legitimately feel it was quite appropriate to recommend additional services as long as they provided at least some potential health benefit to the patient. For example, even if a test were unlikely to change the treatment, as long as it carried no physical risk and it offered at least a little information, it would be reasonable to order it. Of course, the fact that the provider might make a profit from the test could have an additional influence on the recommendation. Thus, the reimbursement system was generally designed to encourage the use of more medical care and to provide no restraints on the use of ever more expensive technologies. Throughout the 1970s, the major funding sources, federal and state governments and private employers, complained about rising costs, but did little to alter the system. There are some notable exceptions in the instance of specific state regulatory programmes, but these had little national impact.

The major cost-containment component of the medical care system through the early 1980s was the presence of some cost-sharing for consumers through annual deductibles and co-insurance. Co-payments were generally precluded, however, in Medicaid programmes because the poor were unable to afford them. In most insurance plans sponsored by large employers, coverage and benefits were increasing, while annual deductibles remained at relatively low levels ($50-100 per person per year), which became less and less significant in the context of the rapid inflation of the 1970s. Furthermore, most insurance plans have a cap on co-payments up to a maximum benefit. This means that for a hospital stay, the patient might be responsible for the first $100 as a deductible, and 20% of the remaining bill up to an out-of-pocket payment of $1 000. Thus, the patient was essentially paying 20 cents per dollar for the first $5 000 of care, with everything free afterwards. (Many plans would stop coverage after $100 000 or $1 000 000 in benefits, but these maximums were rarely exceeded.) Since few hospital stays would account for less than $5 000 in total bills, the system essentially levied an almost flat charge for a hospital stay. Thus, the cost-containing incentives for consumers had their primary effect on reducing ambulatory care through deductibles, but there was relatively little influence on the far more expensive hospital care sector (see Newhouse and Schwartz, 1974; Newhouse *et al.*, 1981).

The HMOs financial incentives are quite different from those of the FFS system described above. For HMOs, the profit (or revenue less expenses for not-for-profit plans) is greater if fewer services are provided – almost all HMOs are able to use their fixed pool of funds to cover both physician and hospital expenses. Thus, if physicians order fewer hospitalisations (or substitute a less expensive for a more expensive test), the savings can be shared with the physicians. This, in turn, generates incentives for cost-containing behaviour on the part of the key decision-makers, the physicians. It also allows the HMO to reduce the use of patient co-payments as a method of cost-containment.

With few exceptions, HMOs marketed their plans to employee and union groups as alternatives to the conventional fee-for-service reimbursement insurance plan. Typically, once a year, the employee could choose to enrol in either the HMO or the FFS insurance plan, with the employer or union paying part or all of the premium. If total costs under the two plan were equivalent, given the absence of co-payments in the HMO, along with a generally more comprehensive benefit package (for example, HMOs cover preventive care in contrast to most insurance plans), one would expect the premiums of the HMO to be higher. However, the cost-containing effects of HMOs over time helped reduce costs to the point that HMO premiums became lower than FFS premiums, even though by enrolling in the former, patients also avoided substantial out-of-pocket costs. This switching of relative prices generally helped to further increase HMO market share within the employee group.

It seems that from the patient's perspective, the comparison between the classic PGP-model HMO and the classic FFS reimbursement plan was one of cost versus freedom of choice. The FFS option would typically allow the enrollee to visit any licensed provider in the country. If a patient was dissatisfied with long waits in the office, wanted a more aggressive treatment plan, or was willing to cross the country to see the "top surgeon", the insurer placed no constraints on such "shopping". This behaviour, of course, helped increase the plan's overall costs, but the resulting increases in premiums were shared by all enrollees and often partly or fully absorbed by the employer or union through increases in their annual contribution to the premium. In contrast, the HMO typically offered a much narrower choice of physicians and hospital settings, but at substantially lower cost. While the two types of plans are substitutes for one another (in the sense that HMOs and insurers with FFS reimbursement both offer coverage for medical care), competition was somewhat muted because of the differences in product and the relatively small number of HMOs in any one market area.

The New Economic Environment

By the mid-1980s the medical care environment had changed substantially. Budgetary pressures on the federal and state governments, and international competitive pressures on employers, have led to an increased willingness among almost all important payers for health care to institute major cost-containment initiatives. The implementation in 1983 of the Prospective Payment System (PPS) for hospitals using diagnosis-related groups (DRGs) by Medicare has had several major effects. First, the fixed payment per admission creates incentives for hospitals to identify less expensive methods of treating specific types of cases. The introduction of PPS also had an important psychological effect on physicians and hospitals who began to be convinced that cost-containment was a real and long-term trend in the medical care system, not just a slogan. PPS was designed to affect only the elderly and was expected to shorten hospital stays but possibly increase admissions. However, even before PPS was fully phased in, stays and admissions fell for both the elderly and the non-elderly. At about the same time, private insurers began raising deductibles, thus increasing consumer cost sensitivity (and simultaneously helping to reduce premiums or at least slow their rise). Insurers also began placing more stringent limits on the hospital charges and physician fee levels. More direct cost-containment efforts were also introduced, such as requiring second opinions before certain surgical admissions, and authorising only limited hospital stays unless unexpected problems occur.

These changes in incentives and expectations resulted in declines in hospital use, thus reducing hospital occupancy levels and creating substantial pressures on individual hospital administrators to remain solvent. Physician supply was also increasing (relative to the demand for services) partly because of long-term growth in medical school graduating classes, and partly because of more time available due to the reduction in hospital use. Concern about the current and rapidly growing physician surplus became commonplace among professionals. Both hospitals and physicians recognised that, in the face of limitations on the resources available for medical care, their economic security depended on obtaining increasing shares of the available funds.

Simultaneously, new types of delivery systems were being developed, in part because of legal decisions allowing more direct advertising by health care providers. Physicians and hospitals began to establish free-standing ambulatory surgery centres and urgent care centres to provide easy access to physicians (Trauner et al., 1982). While community hospitals operating on a not-for-profit basis remained the dominant form of hospital ownership, the early 1980s were a period of extraordinary growth and profitability for proprietary hospital chains. The federal government continued to encourage HMOs, but termination of the grant-and-loan programmes made it more difficult for new plans to raise capital unless they were operated on a for-profit basis. New regulations, moreover, promised a substantially increased role for HMOs in providing care on a capitated basis for Medicare and Medicaid beneficiaries. In some states, such as California, Preferred Provider Organisations, or PPOs, developed in which the insurer or the state Medicaid programme selected only certain hospitals and physicians for special contracts (Trauner, 1983; Gabel and Ermann, 1985; Rice et al., 1985). In return for the promise of a larger share of the relevant market, providers would offer PPOs lower fees, and accept more stringent utilisation review. The falling hospital-occupancy rate, and increasing physician surplus during this period, increased providers' willingness to sign such selective contracts.

While it is difficult to know exactly which changes led to what outcomes, there are some fairly clear changes in system performance. Most notably, hospital utilisation has been falling, for both Medicare beneficiaries and privately-insured enrollees. The latter effect led to a marked slowing in the rate of growth in insurance premiums which, in turn, put much more pressure on HMOs to maintain their economic edge. Simultaneously, the number of HMOs has increased, so plans must compete against one another, not just against the FFS option; this makes market segmentation much more difficult. Employers are becoming increasingly concerned about biased selection; some feel that the HMOs attract healthier enrollees, leaving the "high cost" people to the FFS plan – which then both costs the employer more in direct subsidy and increases the funds payable to the HMOs (Luft et al., 1985).

In some areas of the country, the opening of the Medicare and Medicaid market to HMOs has attracted new organisations that are inexperienced in running HMOs but face strong pressures to show a reasonable return on investment. Moreover, unlike the typical yearly "open season" with group marketing, these publicly-financed beneficiaries generally face continuous marketing pressure as individual enrollees. This direct marketing, the older or poorer population, and the absence of employer-benefits counsellors, have combined to create greater opportunities for misunderstandings and biased enrolment. Some widely-publicised cases of unethical marketing, and quality-of-care deficiencies may merely be isolated cases, but comprehensive impartial studies have yet to be done. Finally, the increasingly competitive nature of the overall health-care market makes it more difficult to obtain data from plans for research purposes, for fear it may give others a competitive advantage. Thus, less rather than more useful information about HMO performance is now available even though there are more HMOs and more HMO enrollees than ever before.

These changes in the United States medical-care system in general, and in HMOs in particular, have important implications for the applicability of the HMO concept in other nations. First, it is clearly demonstrated that HMO performance cannot be evaluated independently from the structure of the medical care financing and policy environment. Not only may HMOs perform differently in other countries, they may be quite different in the United States of the 1980s compared to the United States of the 1970s. Second, some features of HMOs have been applied to new organisational forms in the United States, in particular selective contracts with a limited number of physicians and hospitals. This suggests that pieces of the HMO model may be useful even if the whole is not applicable. Third, the role of provider expectations should be carefully examined, especially when one is considering the political difficulties of instituting major changes. While not yet fully understood, the relatively sudden realisation of the "surplus" of physicians and hospitals may have made possible the segmentation of previously united fronts – various subgroups fighting among themselves to maintain their revenues.

Transferability issues

Given the importance of specific social, legal, historical and economic aspects of the medical care environment in the development and performance of medical care delivery systems such as the HMO, it is not reasonable to expect that the typical HMO from the United States could simply be transplanted to another country. Instead, in this section, I will discuss some of the issues that need to be addressed in transferring specific aspects of the HMO concept to other settings. In some instances, real or hypothetical examples will be drawn either from the United States or international experience to illustrate a point. While these examples may make the discussion a bit more concrete, they are not intended as evaluations or interpretations. The aspects to be considered will be grouped as follows: a) the social contract and public risk-taking, b) physician payment alternatives, c) organisational forms, d) reallocating the medical care budget, and e) consumer incentives.

The social contract and public risk-taking

One key difference between the United States and many other developed nations is the role of government in the medical care system. In some countries the notion of a social contract – and the uniform sharing of risk – is deeply engrained and highly valued. While there may be regional inequities in the availability of services, the intent of the system is to equalise access and coverage. A uniform system of entitlements, even if provided through a multitude of independent providers and insurers with identical benefits, has the advantage of political accountability. In the United States, the Medicare system comes the closest to this model. While local fiscal intermediaries are used for the administration of the programme (and the delivery of care is through independent FFS-providers), benefits and coverage are determined nationally and policy-makers can ask whether beneficiaries are receiving services consistent with their legislative intent.

In some ways, the policy debate in the United States surrounding the use of capitated systems for Medicare beneficiaries may exemplify the concerns that would be raised in other settings. The numerous technical issues of how to set the premium or capitation payment to the HMOs are only part of the problem and will be discussed below. Even if the payments could be designed to adjust for risk differences, problems would still remain. With everyone in a single system such as the conventional Medicare programme, beneficiaries are implicitly guaranteed certain services, or at least certain levels of reimbursement. If people are simply offered choices among several health plans, the promise is converted from one of coverage to a fixed amount of money. One reason capitation plans are attractive to payers such as the government or employers is that the financial risk associated with greater than predicted medical care use or price inflation is passed from the payer to the capitated plan. Of course, the plan will not absorb such risk indefinitely; at some point, cost pressures are likely to be translated into service reductions.

In the United States, programmes such as Medicare are often referred to as "uncontrollables" in budgetary discussions: the government simply cannot predict how much medical care will be used by beneficiaries in a year or what costs will be and, therefore, cannot predict how much money will be spent. Instead, beneficiaries are guaranteed certain levels of coverage and various mechanisms are used to control prices and utilisation. When Medicare beneficiaries are enrolled in HMOs, however, the government knows in advance exactly what its outlays will be for the coming year, making planning much simpler. This shifts the financial risk to the provider and the risk of inadequate services to the enrollee (Cantwell, 1986). As long as the proportion of Medicare beneficiaries enrolled in HMOs remains relatively small, the capitation rates can be tied to the "standard" FFS plan (Rossiter, *et al.,* 1990). Thus, as costs for the FFS enrollees rise (with prices increasing due to inflation) and utilisation changes (with new technology), one can argue that the capitation payments based on the FFS costs are reasonable. However, as the proportion of beneficiaries enrolled in the FFS sector becomes smaller and, perhaps, less representative of those enrolled in the HMOs, the FFS costs are no longer a valid standard and the capitation rate is then likely to be tied to some arbitrary index, such as the rate of growth in Gross Domestic Product. If this happens, the capitation programme for Medicare beneficiaries would be transformed from one of guaranteed benefits to one of a dollar allotment which must be weighed against other budgetary needs. On the one hand, some economists argue that medical care should be treated as any other commodity or service and should be evaluated within global budget constraints. On the other hand, policy-makers often hold that medical care is, and should be, different. In fact, the question of whether a publicly-supported medical care programme should guarantee benefits or dollar subsidies is largely a political, rather than an economic issue and thus is well beyond the scope of this paper. It should be recognised, however, that a major shift towards capitated plans instead of guaranteed benefits is likely to raise precisely this question.

Even if HMOs are intended to be small components of a largely traditional FFS system, problems in screening out poor-quality HMOs may arise in public systems. In the United States, employers and unions have the right to choose which of the various health plan options available in the local community they will offer their employees and members. (While a federally-qualified HMO may be able to mandate access to an employer, this does not alter the basic notion.) In its capacity as an agent for the employees or members, the employer or union can exclude plans that do not meet certain performance requirements. The loss of such a contract is not easily contested in court. In contrast, HMOs are typically brought into publicly-funded programmes through standard government contracting procedures, and cannot be easily cut from the list of available options. Thus, the typical lack of flexibility in governmental contracting becomes even more of a problem when the quality of the product is as difficult to measure as is the case with medical care.

Physician Payment Alternatives

A key aspect of the HMO concept is that providers control the entire range of services included within the benefit package. In particular, this means that if expensive hospital use by enrollees is reduced by physician admitting decisions, these funds may be used for ambulatory services or may be shared with physicians. This raises the difficult question of how one can achieve a reduction in the use of expensive services. The complex and highly-technical nature of medical care makes it difficult for non-physicians to undertake what might be called "micro-management". It is generally impossible to set out explicit criteria for whether patients with specific conditions should be hospitalised. Decision analyses of such problems usually abstract from comorbidities and other factors, thus offering general advice, not clear rules. The broad international literature on variations in practice patterns across small geographical areas and individual physicians, however, suggests there is often wide latitude in clinically-acceptable treatment decision. (Wennberg, 1984; Wennberg and Gittelsohn, 1973 and 1982; Wennberg *et al.,* 1980; see also, Copenhagen Collaborating Center, 1986). The existence of such "grey areas" within which equally competent physicians can disagree on appropriate treatment, offers the opportunity to encourage more conservative practice styles by HMO physicians through alteration of the standard economic incentives.

It may be useful to begin by considering the incentives under various payment systems. FFS payment gives the physician the strongest incentives to offer more services and minimises the physician's financial risk associated with a patient requiring additional care. At the other extreme, pure salary arrangements offer the physician the least incentive for increased productivity, and even cost-containment becomes irrelevant. Capitation creates incentives to add patients to the provider's list, while minimising the provision of services to those within the capitation pool. Thus, if a physician is capitated just for primary care, there are incentives to refer the "troublesome" patient to specialists because those costs are not borne by the primary care physician, or to encourage that patient to join another physician's pool. On the other hand, placing the primary care physician fully at risk for referral services, and perhaps even the associated hospital costs, can create substantial problems. While there is often considerable discretion in determining the need for hospitalisation, a typical individual physician's panel of capitated patients is usually so small that the random occurrence of a few patients who need expensive services can deplete the physician's entire risk pool even if the physician is a frugal user of resources.

Thus it seems best to make capitation payments to groups of physicians who share in the gains or losses. The number of physicians in the pool should be large enough so that random fluctuation in patients' health status average out, yet small enough so that an individual physician can recognise some rewards for more conservative practice. Modifications also can be made to such a plan. For example, the risk of patient care needs for hospitalisation can be borne through risk-pooling with larger groups of physicians while the risk for primary care services might be borne by individual physicians. Throughout the development of such risk pools, one should be searching for the correct balance of incentives to reward cost-effective decision-making by physicians while not imposing unreasonable risks for either physician or patient. Thus, the incentives should encourage more cautious use of expensive resources within the "grey area" reflecting the appropriate range of clinical alternatives, but not push physicians to constrain resource use so severely that the level of care is unacceptable low.

To the extent that HMOs are designed to help reduce the use of expensive medical care, one must incorporate both the primary-care physician and the specialist. Their roles in the United States differ from those in many other developed nations. This difference can have an important impact on the design of capitation plans. In the United States, the patient with FFS insurance coverage typically has free access to both primary-care physicians and specialists. Both make treatment decisions, bill patients, and run their medical practices independently in the United States as well. The major difference for hospital-based specialties such as anaesthesiology, pathology, and radiology is that they rarely decide whether a treatment or test is to be performed, but most are quite independent of the hospital in which they practise. Thus, one can identify three groups of decision-makers:

a) Primary-care physicians who can follow their patients and provide many types of general medical and surgical care in the hospital;
b) Specialists who advise on whether certain types of special services should be rendered, often by themselves and the hospital; and
c) Hospitals and hospital-based physicians whose responsibility is the provision of specialised services generally prescribed by physicians in the first two categories.

The last group of physicians generally has incentives for developing productivity-enhancing technology even within the FFS system and these incentives will become even stronger with the Prospective Payment System. It is important, however, to distinguish incentives to reduce the cost of providing specific services, from the incentives to order fewer services. Capitated plans such as HMOs will often contract with hospitals in ways that create incentives for the hospitals to be efficient providers of service, but may not hold them responsible for the number of services ordered. Instead, incentives to constrain the number of services ordered have to be focused on the first two groups of decision-makers.

In the United States, there is a highly complex but not well understood system of referral patterns among primary-care and specialist physicians. Referrals in both directions are commonplace because many specialists also serve as generalists. Because it is illegal to split fees to induce referrals, physicians cultivate referral relationships in more informal ways. One aspect of the relationship is the shared responsibility of primary-care and specialist physician for in-patient care. This shared responsibility and close working relationship probably lead to an intuitive sense of differences in practice styles among various physicians. For example, there is some evidence that the existing referral system tends to channel patients towards those hospitals and specialists with better-than-average outcomes, even though explicit outcome statistics are not readily available (Luft *et al.,* 1987; Luft *et al.,* 1990). In many other countries, there is a sharp distinction between the primary-care physician (whose responsibility ends at the hospital door) and the specialist who a) is responsible for all hospital care, b) may be paid on an entirely different basis, and c) may have a different career path. The shared responsibility of generalist and specialist in the United States may or may not be a crucial aspect of the HMO model, but it is probably not irrelevant. Clearly, if specialists have no cost-containing incentives, then some of the largest potential savings may be overlooked. This suggests that physician payment alternatives have to be integrated into an overall organisational design which includes both primary-care physicians and specialists.

In nations with clear divisions between primary-care physicians and salaried hospital specialists, it is more difficult to import the classic United States HMO with its single pool of specialists and generalists. There are, however, some United States HMOs that have developed in such environments. For example, most medical school faculties are on something similar to a salary arrangement; even if they bill patients on a fee-for-service basis, the fees are often turned over to the department, which may be more willing to agree to future salary increases if revenues are high. Some medical school-based HMOs are formed around a central core of primary-care physicians who then refer to specialists in other departments in the medical school when appropriate. The HMO patients may represent all or a major share of the sub-specialist's practice. The specialty departments may be paid on a fee-for-service basis by the HMO (but recall that the HMO controls access to the specialist) or the HMO may use a capitation rate for the department, e.g., X-$ per enrollee per year to cover all neurosurgical care. The sub-specialists may still want to practise high technology style medicine and, unless paid on a capitation basis, they have no direct incentive to do otherwise. The primary-care physicians, however, would monitor the use of services by specific specialists and attempt to direct referrals towards those who are more conservative.

Any innovation requires overcoming resistance to change in traditional modes of behaviour. One way to accomplish this is to provide incentives for the potential participants. Thus, even if faculty physicians are paid on a strict salary basis, there is generally the expectation that if the new HMO arrangement works, a) salaries might be increased, b) there may be bonuses, c) the department chair will have funds available for professional meetings, or d) the benefits will, in some other way, be at least partially shared. Sometimes the incentive is not the addition of benefits, but a chance to maintain one's position in the face of declining budgets. Without some flexibility, however, the chances of success are greatly reduced.

Organisational forms

In the United States, the HMO economic incentives have been applied to different types of organisations. The PGP-model HMO has provided the best evidence of cost-containing ability with reasonable quality. Some IPA models with networks of physician groups show similar performance, even if those groups originally focused on, and still primarily serve, FFS patients. HMOs with an IPA model having more loosely associated physicians demonstrate a wider range of costs and medical care utilisation. There are several potential explanations for these differences. The formation of a medical group, be it FFS or capitated, may make it easier for generalists and specialists to develop consistent modus operandi and become comfortable with a particular practice style. By working together, they get to know one another's abilities, they can consult informally, and they do not need to fear the potential loss of patients to others within the group. The group also provides a natural risk pool for capitation payments – large enough to avoid some of the problems associated with capitation for individual physicians, while still allowing the inclusion of hospital and specialist services.

The work setting of both FFS and prepaid multispecialty groups may also tend to attract less individualistic physicians comfortable with some type of income-sharing. This means that physicians who would tend to earn less in solo FFS practice (such as paediatricians), earn more in a group setting, while others (such as surgeons) earn less in groups than they would in solo practice. A group setting also allows physicians a somewhat different "life style" than solo practice, with less individual responsibility for "on-call" time, less control over one's own schedule and work environment, and more free time. These characteristics of group practice may help attract physicians who are more conservative users of medical care. On the other hand, there is increasing evidence that some IPAs which do not use groups are also able to control costs, but it seems they tend to use more direct controls over utilisation, rather than the more implicit rules found in groups (Hillman et al., 1989).

Thus, the implementation of a capitation approach in other countries may depend on what practice models already exist. If multispecialty groups or clinics are present, it may be possible to establish

54

capitation contracts with these organisations, allowing the physicians and clinic administrators to develop their own schemes for the division of the fund pool. (It is noteworthy that the methods for dividing the available pool among physicians within groups is one of the most closely guarded secrets of HMOs.) If such organisations are not already present, then analogues will have to be developed, although it may well be possible to have an "HMO without walls", in which physicians do not practise together, but merely form an economically-related group. The development of such a group needs attention since one would like to attract only those physicians comfortable with the HMO style of practice and organisation.

The financial incentives of the HMO may have little to do with its cost-containing performance. Instead, they may merely serve to attract physicians with more conservative practice styles. (As an analogy, the faculties of business schools are less likely than are small "start-up firms" to attract professionals who are risk-takers.) New HMOs in an environment in which they are not well-understood will have to design the appropriate set of signals to attract the "correct" types of physicians. For example, an emphasis on HMOs as a means whereby physicians are able to exercise more professional autonomy (without external bureaucratic controls and bothersome paperwork, as long as their subsystem remains within budget) is likely to attract rather different types of physicians than an emphasis on HMOs as a means of increasing profits while containing costs. Thus, it is crucial that one keeps in mind the interplay between the role of incentives in shaping behaviour and the selection of individuals comfortable with those incentives.

This raises questions of organisational sponsorship and goals. If the only funds available for start-up costs and experimentation come from private sources, then there will be a greater expectation of the system returning a profit in the short run. On the other hand, public agencies, at least in the United States, have rarely been willing to establish their own HMO systems; the risk of failure is substantial, and the rewards are far less clear to the public decision-maker. Public support has been available, however, in the form of grants and loans to non-profit HMOs which then allow the development of systems with less focus on profitability. Mixed public-private or semi-autonomous enterprises outside the government bureaucracy are also a possible selection. The organisation is then one in which the government is the prime or sole shareholder.

Reallocating the medical care budget

The underlying attraction of HMOs is the notion that key decision-makers (such as physicians) can be attracted to the HMO by the promise of increased personal incomes while, at the same time, the total cost of care is reduced. The obvious way this is achieved is by reallocating the shares of a smaller pie, often by reducing hospital use. Since expenditures in a sector are the source of income for workers in that sector, this implies a reduction in hospital use and staffing. It may also imply a relative shift of expenditures on physician services away from in-patient-oriented specialists towards primary-care physicians and, more importantly, those physicians working in HMO settings. In some nations, the political implications of such shifts may be substantial.

Politics aside, the mechanics of the shift may be difficult in some systems, especially those in which the financing systems for physicians, in particular primary-care physicians, and in-patient care are separate. This may be seen through a brief discussion of the Kaiser-Permanente HMO system, the largest in the United States. The Kaiser Foundation Health Plan is the formal HMO organisation. It enrols members for a fixed premium and promises the necessary medical care will be made available. To do this, it contracts with the Permanent Medical Group, a legally separate (but closely related) physician partnership, to provide the necessary physician services on a capitation basis. The Health Plan also contracts with Kaiser Foundation Hospitals for hospital care based on the expected number of enrollees. If less hospital care is used than anticipated in the contract, the savings are split between the Kaiser Foundation Hospitals and the Permanente Medical Group. In order to remain competitive in the health insurance market, the Health Plan attempts to minimise its payments to the other two groups. Over time, as Kaiser physicians have developed ways of caring for their patients with fewer hospital days, the hospital's share of the total pie has fallen, but in absolute terms, enrolment growth allows for hospital expansion.

If there were no way to shift funds from the hospital side to the physician side, then it would be difficult to reward the clinical decision-makers for the development of more cost-effective practice styles. There need not be formal contractual connections between the HMO and hospitals for these shifts to occur. Most HMOs do not own their own hospitals but, instead, pay for the care of their patients in various ways similar to those used by conventional insurers. (In some cases this includes discounts to reflect bargaining power or efficiencies in group purchasing and payment.) If the HMO physicians request less hospital care for their patients, however, there is more money left for the HMO to spend elsewhere, such as the physician pool.

If the HMO has no responsibility for paying for hospital care (perhaps because it is covered by an entirely separate agency, as in many other countries) then it cannot appropriate the savings unless other arrangements are made. Indeed, an HMO in such a system has incentives to shift costs the other way, substituting expensive hospital care (for which it has no responsibility) for less expensive ambulatory care covered in its capitation payment. For example, suppose that people are universally covered by both a hospital insurance plan (paid for by the State) and by a separate set of physician insurance plans for which there is some consumer cost. In such a system, there is no direct linkage between the two plans and, if the physician insurers were to develop incentives for their physicians to order less hospital care, the State would be the prime beneficiary – this would reduce the incentive for the insurers to undertake such a risky innovation. To encourage such behaviour, however, the state hospital plan might estimate the number of hospital days that would usually be required (per thousand covered individuals, per year) and then track the actual use of people enrolled in the new system. If their subsequent use is actually lower than the average, some of the implicit savings might be shared with the physician insurance plan which, in turn, could use the funds to *a)* reward their physicians, *b)* lower premiums, or *c)* increase benefits.

A key aspect of any set of contractual relationships, such as is implicit in the HMO model, is the expectation by each party that they will be better off under the new arrangement than under the old. Under this premise, one should ask whether the approach outlined above for sharing funds between the hypothetical government-sponsored hospital funds and the physician insurers is sufficient. If it is compared to the Kaiser model, it is immediately apparent that no incentives have been included for the hospitals. Suppose that the hospitals in the existing system operate under a budget set by the Health Ministry. If patient days fall because of the HMO incentives, the Ministry can achieve savings to share with the HMO by reducing the hospital's budget. (If the budget is not reduced even when occupancy falls, then the introduction of the HMO actually costs the Ministry money.) The hospital administrator probably has numerous potential methods available for maintaining occupancy levels, and these are all the more powerful if in-patient specialist physicians also have an interest in maintaining their patient load. However, just as a plan could be developed to estimate and share with the primary-care physicians the savings attributable to lower hospital use, some of those savings could be shared with the "contracting" hospitals. Of course, political problems could arise from what appears to be paying hospitals to have no patients, but this is just one aspect of the reversal of incentives in capitated plans.

The appropriate design of incentives for the various parties that must participate in the HMO is further complicated by the often mixed public-private nature of health-care providers. In many countries, hospitals are primarily publicly owned, while physicians (and sometimes insurers) are in the private sector. As long as the payments to hospitals on the one hand, and to physicians on the other, remain separate, then few problems occur. However, designing an HMO which reallocates funds between the two groups raises political and legal problems that are far more important than the simple design of economic incentives. For example, public hospitals which are accustomed to having an overall budget constraint may have no basis upon which they can set contractual prices for the care of HMO patients. Without some reasonably objective method of determining the savings attributable to the reduced hospital use of the HMO members, the stage is set for conflict – not only between the HMO and the hospital, but between FFS providers and state hospitals. This again raises the issue of whether the new plans should be public, private, or have a mixed sponsorship. Even a public system is not above controversy, as may be seen whenever one government agency attempts to charge another for services rendered.

Another issue that must be addressed in the context of "dividing the pie" is that of selective contracting. By their nature, HMOs include only some of the potentially available physicians and hospitals in the local area. This allows the smaller number of providers to increase their individual revenue while at the same time reducing overall expenses. For example, suppose that under a FFS system orthopaedists developed fairly broad indications for back surgery, and this allowed 100 surgeons to be fully occupied caring for the problems occurring in a population of 1 000 000. It may be the case that more conservative treatment regimens could care for the same number of people with half the amount of surgery, albeit with more physical therapy. An HMO covering half that population might seek to include only 25 orthopaedists so that each could be fully occupied, with no reduction in income, but far less would be spent on orthopaedic surgery overall. However, this arrangement leaves

75 orthopaedists scrambling to support themselves on a population base that previously supported 50 of them.

Of course, any arrangement of this type implies inclusion of some providers and exclusion of others. This is not only likely to raise political hackles, but poses problems of implementation as well. Voluntary co-operation is generally desirable, especially if the correct incentives can be designed to attract the appropriate physicians. For example, if office-based physicians are currently paid primarily on a FFS basis, those more inclined to provide tests and procedures often earn higher incomes, while those who spend more time with the patient discussing their problems, and are more conservative in their ordering patterns, earn less. A capitated system, with its incentives to reduce the use of marginally necessary services, represents quite a shift in practice patterns for the first type of physician and less of a change for the second. Capitation is also less likely to offer the same level of income for the second. An open invitation for physicians to join the HMO may thus attract primarily the second type of physician, which is a desirable outcome from the perspective of the HMO. It uses the differences in economic incentives in the two systems to attract selectively those physicians who will be most comfortable in each system.

While the HMO may be able to maintain or increase the income of its practitioner members, the shift of patients into the HMO implies lower patient loads for those physicians not in the system. Increased competition among the remaining FFS providers for a shrinking patient pool is likely to produce political opposition to the HMOs. Such opposition may well focus on the incentives of the HMO to undertreat its enrollees, and may even use the preference of HMO physicians for less aggressive practice patterns as "evidence of their poor quality". Thus, it is important that strategies to implement HMOs incorporate carefully-designed systems to monitor quality. Quality measures can focus both on process or outcome (see Donabedian, 1968, for the classic discussion of quality assessment). Process measures concentrate on whether the appropriate actions were taken for a patient with a particular problem, such as the prescription of antihypertensive medication for a patient with high blood pressure. Outcome measures can focus on either mortality, such as the death rate due to stroke or hypertensive heart disease in comparable populations, or morbidity, such as the extent of uncontrolled hypertension in the patient population. There are advantages and disadvantages to each type of quality assessment measure when comparing delivery systems and a combination of both approaches is probably the best strategy (Luft, 1981).

Consumer incentives

To provide genuine choice to the consumer, the design of any alternative care financing and delivery system must necessarily include incentives for both the user and the provider. The question of choice is an important one, and it may well be the case that a unitary system is preferable for political or other reasons. A system that offers a choice among plans has the advantage of an inherent competitive pressure continually to improve service. Such pressures may prove more effective than traditional budgetary pressure where evaluation of outcomes is difficult. Offering various delivery systems also reduces the political opposition to a forced transfer of the public into a new system. Instead, people choose the new system only if it appears to be advantageous to them. However, making available a choice of plans also creates several important problems which will be discussed below.

Consumers may be offered various incentives to enrol in HMOs or alternative delivery systems. In the United States, HMOs generally offer a more comprehensive range of benefits than do the conventional plans, and thus cover a wide range of preventive services and prescription drugs not usually offered by insurance plans. The HMOs also usually eliminate the use of deductibles and have only minimal co-payments, so the lack of financial barriers can be an incentive. Finally, this package of benefits and coverage is frequently available at a lower monthly premium than the conventional FFS insurance plan. Since HMOs generally offer a more constrained practice style and sometimes have non-financial barriers to care (such as longer waits for an appointment and less continuity of care with the same physician), these negatives must be weighed by consumers and balanced against lower overall cost.

Different types of trade-offs are possible in various countries. For example, some European countries have mixed insurance systems in which the worker is partly responsible for the health insurance premium. In such cases, the HMO could attract enrollees by offering a lower premium for comparable coverage. If the employer is responsible for the direct payment of the premium, the situation is a bit more complex. The employer can save money only if workers are encouraged to enrol in the HMO. Employees may be given incentives to enrol in the HMO through bonuses equal to the premium savings or the purchase of additional benefits, such as dental coverage if that is not readily available.

It may be the case that the existing system offers few options for additional financial incentives because it already provides comprehensive coverage with no patient co-payments or premiums. Such a system implies an external source of funding which is likely to impose other kinds of constraints to stay within budgetary limits. Suppose that these constraints operate through restrictions on the number of physicians, or have the effect of limiting the amount of personal care offered by the hospital staff. An HMO might attract enrollees by enhancing the availability of primary care physicians so that patients are able to obtain appointments on short notice or find such appointments easily available on evenings and weekends. Similarly, the HMO might develop the reputation for having the best hospital food and most attentive nurses. As long as its physicians are able to constrain the use of expensive services below that of the competing conventional system, the added costs can be absorbed by the system and may serve as incentives for consumers to enrol in the plan.

While it may be quite important that there be competition between the conventional system (whatever it is), and the new alternative delivery system, it is less clear that there must be several alternative delivery systems in a local area. The major HMOs in the United States, such as Kaiser and Group Health Cooperative, developed quite effective cost-containment systems with little competition in their local areas from other HMOs. It is even possible that the potential market for HMOs, given their distinctive delivery system, is limited to substantially less than the total population and vigorous local competition merely leads to costly advertising and contention over market share without increased system-wide efficiency.

One of the problems associated with vigorous local competition among HMOs is that it may be far easier to keep costs below a fixed capitation level through favourable risk selection than through cost-effective provision of services. Thus, competition among local HMOs may encourage them to attract those people who are least likely to use medical care while devising ways to avoid enrolling those people most in need of services. Some biased selection is natural, based upon the location of the various service delivery sites, the reputation of the providers, and differences in benefit packages. The United States' Medicare programme has developed a fairly complex set of risk categories to compute a risk-adjusted premium for HMOs serving Medicare beneficiaries on a capitated basis, but some analysts still feel there is substantial leeway for selection (Gruenberg et al., 1986). It is likely that the problems of biased selection are reduced if the system has yearly rather than monthly open enrolment seasons during which people can change plans. Selection may also be reduced if there is no direct contact between the plans and potential enrollees during marketing; instead, materials should be provided through an intermediary such as an employer or union (Enthoven, 1986). It may be necessary to adopt more complex methods of monitoring and adjusting for selective biases if these relatively simple approaches fail to reduce the differences across plans to a tolerable level (Luft, 1985; Robinson et al., 1991). Some argue, however, that complete adjustment for biased selection is impossible (Jones, 1989).

In any event, there are two basic notions that must be remembered when dealing with biased selection in the context of capitated plans. The first is that plans have an incentive to avoid enrolling individuals they feel will be more costly than the associated capitation payment. This need not imply that HMOs will only be willing to accept the healthiest enrollees. On the contrary, if capitation payments are made on a risk-adjusted basis, there are far greater savings to be made for someone likely to have expensive illnesses that can be treated in various ways, such as AIDS, than for someone expected to be healthy whose only need for care is the small probability of an accident. The key is to adjust the capitation rate up or down to reflect the enrollee's risk factors. The second point is that while the plan should be paid more for a high-risk enrollee, the additional cost of the higher premium payment to the plan should be borne socially, rather than by the victim. The patient's share should only reflect differences in the efficiency of the alternative delivery systems after risk factors have been taken into account.

Conclusions

There is substantial evidence that in the relatively non-competitive medical care environment of the United States up to the early 1980s, many HMOs were able to provide care for their enrollees at substantially lower cost than the conventional FFS. While this often involved various types of access barriers, HMOs removed financial barriers to care, and the quality of services was comparable to that offered in the conventional system. It is not yet clear whether the same type of performance continued since, in a more competitive and cost-conscious environment.

Since the HMO is really a combination of organisations of providers and a system of economic incentives, its performance is strongly influenced by its social, economic, legal, and political environment. Rather than a broad-spectrum antibiotic, which is likely to work against a wide range of infections and whose efficacy is assured by simple manufacturing processes, HMOs are more like a complex surgical technique, in which one must make sure that the surgeon is carefully trained and, furthermore, that the technique is appropriate for the patient's specific problem. Even in the United States in a given time period, various HMOs perform differently. When considering their applicability to other nations, one should first inquire as to what is the perceived local problem before reaching for the HMO model as a solution. Once the problem is understood, it may be far better to consider the HMO not as a "package" to be imported, but as a set of lessons concerning the use of incentives to shape medical care delivery. Viewed in this way, one may be able to examine which aspects of HMOs may be useful in a restructuring of the medical care system to achieve the desired goals. In doing so, however, one should keep in mind that our understanding of how the medical system works is far from complete, so newly developed models are unlikely to work exactly as planned. Each new model should teach us about the system and help in the creation of yet better alternatives.

Bibliography

Burns, L.R. and Wholey, D.R. (1991), "Differences in access and qualiy of care across HMO types", *Health Services Management Research,* March, pp. 32-45.

Cantwell, J.R. (1986), "Are Capitation Levels Under or Over Compensating Medicare Risk HMOS?", US General Accounting Office, Paper presented at the Annual Meetings of the Western Economic Association, San Francisco, July 1.

Copenhagen Collaborating Center for the Study of Regional Variations in Health Care (1986), *CCC Bibliography on Regional Variations in Health Care 1985,* Copenhagen.

Cunningham, F.C. and Williamson, J.W. (1880), "How Does the Quality of Health Care in HMOs Compare to That in Other Settings? An Analytical Literature Review: 1958 to 1979", *The Group Health Journal,* I, Winter, pp. 4-25.

Donabedian, A. (1968), *Medical Care Appraisal: Quality and Appraisal,* New York, American Public Health Association.

Donabedian, A. (1978), "The Quality of Medical Care", *Science,* 200, May 26, pp. 856-858.

Enthoven, A.C. (1986), "Managed Competition and the Unfinished Agenda for Competition in Health Care", Graduate School of Business, Stanford University, August.

Gabel, J. and Ermann, D. (1985), "Preferred Provider Organizations: Performance, Problems and Promise", *Health Affairs,* 4:1, Spring, pp. 24-40.

Gruenberg, L., Wallack, S.S. and Tomkins, Ch.P. (1986), "Pricing Strategies for Capitated Delivery Systems", Health Policy Center, Heller Graduate School, Brandeis University, August.

Hellinger, F.J. (1987), "Selection bias in health maintenance organizations: analysis of recent evidence", *Health Care Financing Review,* 9:2, Winter, pp. 55-63.

Hillman, A.L., Pauly, M.V. and Kerstein, J.J. (1989), "How do financial incentives affect physicians' clinical decisions and the financial performance of health maintenance organizations?", *New England Journal of Medicine,* 321:2, pp. 86-92.

Jones, S.B. (1989), "Can multiple choice be managed to contain health care costs?", *Health Affairs,* 8:3, Fall, pp. 51-59.

Luft, H.S. (1980a), "Trends in Medical Care Costs: Do HMOs Lower the Rate of Growth?", *Medical Care,* 18:1, January 1, pp. 1-16.

Luft, H.S. (1980b), "The Relation Between Surgical Volume and Mortality: An Exploration of Causal Factors and Alternative Models", *Medical Care,* 18:9, September, pp. 940-959.

Luft, H.S. (1981), *Health Maintenance Organizations: Dimensions of Performance,* New York, Wiley – Interscience.

Luft, H.S. (1985), "Compensating for Biased Selection in Health Insurance", *Millbank Quarterly,* pp. 566-592.

Luft, H.S. (1987), *Health Maintenance Organizations: Dimensions of Performance,* New Brunswick, N.J., Transation Books.

Luft, H.S. and Crane, S. (1980), "Regionalization of Services within a Multihospital Health Maintenance Organization", *Health Services Research,* 15:3, Fall, pp. 231-247.

Luft, H.S., Garnick, D.W., Mark, D.H., Peltzman, D.J., Phibbs, C.S., Lichtenberg, E. and McPhee, S.J. (1990), "Does quality influence choice of hospital?", *Journal of the American Medical Association* 263:21, 6 June, pp. 2899-2906.

Luft, H.S., Hunt, S.S. and Maerki, S.C. (1987), "The volume-outcome relationship: practice makes perfect or selective referral patterns?", *Health Services Research,* 22:2, June, pp. 157-182.

Luft, H.S., Maerki, S.C. and Trauner, J.B. (1986), "Competitive Effects of Health Maintenance Organizations: Another Look at the Evidence from Hawaii, Rochester, N.Y., and Minneapolis-St. Paul", *Journal of Health Politics Policy and Law,* 10:4, Winter, pp. 625-658.

Luft, H.S. and Miller, R.H. (1988), "Patient selection in a competitive health care system", *Health Affairs,* 7:3, Summer, pp. 97-119.

Luft, H.S., Trauner, J.B. and Maerki, S.C. (1985), "Adverse Selection in a Large, Multiple-Option Health Benefits Program: A Case Study of the California Public Employees' Retirement System", in *Advances in Health Economics and Health Services Research,* R.M. Scheffler and L.F. Rossiter (eds.), Greenwich Conn., JAI Press Inc., pp. 197-229.

Manning, W.G., Liebowitz, A., Goldberg, G.A. *et al.* (1984), "A Controlled Trial of the Effect of a Prepaid Group Practice on Use of Services", *New England Journal of Medicine,* 310(23), June 7, pp. 1505-10.

McLaughlin, C.G., Merrill, J.C. and Freed, A.J. (1984), "The Impact of HMO Growth on Hospital Costs and Utilization", in *Advances in Health Economics and Health Services Research,* Vol. 5, Greenwich Conn., JAI Press.

Morrison, E.M. and Luft, H.S. (1990), "HMO environments in the 1980s and beyond", *Healh Care Financing Review,* 12:1, Fall, pp. 81-90.

Newhouse, J.P. and Schwartz, W.B. (1974), "Policy Options and the Impact of National Health Insurance", *New England Journal of Medicine,* 290:24, June 13, pp. 1345-1359.

Newhouse, J.P., Manning, W.G., Morris, C. *et al.* (1981), "Some Interim Results from a Controlled Trial of Cost Sharing in Health Insurance", *New England Journal of Medicine,* 305:25, December 17, pp. 1501-1507.

Newhouse, J.P., Schwartz, W.B., Williams, A.R. and Witsberger, Ch., (1985), "Are Fee-For-Service Costs Increasing Faster Than HMO Costs?", *Medical Care,* 23:8, August, pp. 960-966.

Rice, T., de Lissovoy, G., Gabel, J. and Ermann, D. (1985), "The State of Preferred Provider Organizations: A National Survey", *Health Affairs,* 4:4, Winter, pp. 5-40.

Robinson, J.C., Luft, H.S., Gardner, L.B. and Morrison, E.M.A. (1991), "Method for risk-adjusting employer contributions to competing health insurance plans", *Inquiry,* 28:2, Summer), pp. 107-116.

Rossiter, L.F., Adamche, K.W. and Faulknier, T. (1990), "A blended sector rate adjustment for the Medicare AAPCC when risk-based market penetrion is high", *Journal of Risk and Insurance,* 57:2, June, pp. 220-239.

Trauner, J.B. (1983), "Preferred Provider Organizations: The California Experiment", Institute for Health Policy Studies, University of California, San Francisco, August.

Trauner, J.B., Luft, H.S. and Robinson, J.0. (1982), *Entrepreneurial Trends in Health Care Delivery: The Development of Retail Dentistry and Freestanding Ambulatory Services,* Washington, D.C., Federal Trade Commission, July.

Ware, J.E. *et al.* (1986), "Comparison of Health Outcomes at a Health Maintenance Organization with Those of Fee-For-Service Care", *The Lancet,* May 3, pp. 1017-1022.

Wennberg, J.E. (1984), "Dealing with Medical Practice Variations: A Proposal for Action", *Health Affairs,* 3:2, Summer, pp. 6-32.

Wennberg, J.E. and Gittelsohn, A. (1973), "Small Area Variations in Health Care Delivery", *Science,* 182:4117, 14 December, pp. 1102-08.

Wennberg, J.E. and Gittelsohn, A. (1982), "Variations in Medical Care Among Small Areas", *Scientific American,* 246:4, April.

Wennberg, J.E., Bunker, J.P. and Barnes, B. (1980), "The Need for Assessing the Outcome of Common Clinical Practices", *Annual Review of Public Health,* 1, pp. 277-95.

Wilensky, G.R. and Rossiter, L.F. (1983), "The Relative Importance of Physician-induced Demand in the Demand for Medical Care", *Milbank Memorial Fund Quarterly/Health and Society,* 61:2, pp. 252-277.

Wolinsky, F.D. (1980), "The Performance of HMOS: An Analytic Review", *Milbank Quarterly,* 58:4, Fall, pp. 537-587.

EVALUATION OF COST-CONTAINMENT ACTS IN GERMANY

by

Markus Schneider

Since 1977, cost containment has been an integral part of health policy in the Federal Republic of Germany. The common goal of the cost-containment acts was to bring the growth of health care expenditures in line with wage growth and salaries of sickness-fund members. The Health Care Structure Act of 1993 is the most recent manifestation of this policy. The main features of the numerous cost-containment acts are described in this article, and their effects on demand and supply are analysed.

From 1980 to 1990 the share of gross domestic product (GDP) devoted to health care decreased in the former Federal Republic of Germany from 8.4 to 8.1%. This decrease is opposite to developments in most other Western countries. In the United States, for example, the share of GDP devoted to health care increased from 9.3 to 12.4%. In France, the increase was 1.3% for the same period, and in Canada 1.6% (*OECD Health Data,* 1991). Therefore, cost-containment policy in Germany seems to have been more successful than in many other OECD countries.

Following a short description of some special features of the health care system, is an overview of both health expenditures and various cost-containment measures taken since 1977. Two questions are addressed. Why is cost containment successful? What are the economic results of the cost-containment measures?

The German Health Care System

Although the history of the sickness funds in Germany dates back to the Middle Ages, the foundation of the modern health care system was laid by Bismarck in 1883 (Rosenberg, 1986). The government requires that working persons have compulsory health insurance, regardless of their income. For both blue- and white-collar workers, contributions are calculated as a percentage of gross wages up to an income ceiling. This ceiling determines the maximum contribution. The contributions are collected monthly as a payroll tax from the employers. However, the full cost of the contribution is split 50-50 between employer and employee.

There are several sickness funds providing what is called "social health insurance". At present, these include 259 local sickness funds, 680 company sickness funds, 148 guild sickness funds, 19 agricultural sickness funds, one seamen's and one miners' sickness fund, and 15 substitute ones. In these 1 123 sickness funds about 88% of the total population are insured, about 75% thereof compulsorily. All employees under income limit, unemployed persons, pensioners, self-employed farmers, disabled persons, students and artists are covered by social sickness funds.

It is worth noting that of the insured people free to choose either private insurance or social funds, the majority choose the latter. There is a simple reason for this. In most cases, for married couples and families with children, the premiums of private insurance companies are higher than sickness fund contributions. As a consequence, there is risk selection between sickness funds and private insurance companies. Single persons, with incomes above the compulsory-insurance income ceiling, prefer private insurance companies. Families more frequently choose to be insured by social sickness funds.

Compared with other countries, the most significant characteristic of the German system is the organisation of sickness-fund physicians under public law. There are *Länder* organisations of sickness-fund physicians (for ambulatory care), 19 of which are for physicians and 17 for dentists. These organisations control both the regional access of physicians to provide ambulatory care for patients of social sickness funds, and the reimbursement of fees. Quarterly, each office-based physician sends the vouchers for patients of the sickness funds to the regional organisation for reimbursement. The organisation itself monitors the volume and value of services of each physician. Furthermore, the organisation controls the number and value of prescriptions and referrals. Therefore, these organisations of sickness-fund physicians play an important role in the cost-containment process.

Corresponding to the *Länder* organisations of sickness-fund physicians are the *Länder* associations of the sickness funds. There are general contracts at federal and *Land* levels for the delivering and monitoring of medical services. These general contracts regulate the particulars of the medical services rendered, principles of reimbursement, fees for services, processing of claims, and economic monitoring. These contracts provide the general public framework (without direct involvement of the government) for the relationships between the sickness funds and the sickness-fund physicians.

This self-regulation by the associations of funds and organisations of physicians is a central principle of the German social health system since the beginning of the last century (Herder-Dorneich, 1980). Although the principle of self-regulation is not indisputable, it is not generally questioned from a general point of view because of the political power of the health care administrations. All cost-containment acts in Germany emphasize the importance of the principle of self-regulation. Nevertheless, the cost-containment acts define the obligations of the health care organisations quite specifically. The administrations of these organisations are obliged to promote cost effectiveness, and to align the increase of health expenditures with income.

Institutions comparable to the organisations of sickness-fund physicians do not exist in the hospital area. The 3 000 hospitals negotiate directly with the sickness funds. Consequently, the institutional framework of the hospital requires other measures of cost-containment than the ambulatory area. Furthermore, there is another reason why cost containment for hospital services requires a different concept. Hospital investments are financed by the *Länder,* current expenditures by the sickness funds. This dual financing system promotes numerous conflicts of interest.

Development of health expenditures

Prior to 1977

After the Second World War, the expenditures of the social sickness funds were at a low level. As the economy in Germany started to grow, contributions to the sickness funds increased. This increase, in combination with legislation making more services available to insured members, caused expenditures to raise. This legislatively-mandated expansion required a steady increase of financial contributions by employees and employers. During the period 1950-1960, the expenditures of the sickness funds increased at an annual rate of about 16%. Many warnings concerning the ultimate effect of this rate of increase went unheeded, mainly because of economic prosperity. During the 1960s health expenditures increased, on the average, at an annual rate of about 10%, increasing to some 20% from 1971 to 1975, making this cost explosion a major public and political concern.

At this time, a projection of future health expenditures was published. Geißler, the former Minister of Social Affairs in the Rhineland-Palatinate *Land* forecasted (by trend extrapolation) that, with continued high growth rates for health care expenditures, by the year 2000 one-half of the GNP would be spent on health. He called for action (Geißler, 1976), and thus began a debate on cost containment in the sickness-fund system.

In 1975, the unemployment rate increased to 4.8%, the highest since 1955. The German economy was in the midst of a recession. The rate of return on capital fell to 1.3%. Comparably low capital return rates followed in 1982 and 1983. The recession enforced the pressure to reduce health care costs. Public discussions on cost trends and alternative cost-containment activities – such as a common national sickness fund – led to the voluntary agreement between sickness funds and the organisations of sickness-fund physicians to restrict the increase of global compensations for office-based services. The national organisations of both contracting parties made recommendations to their respective organisations at the *Land* level (Figure 1) to limit the increase. As a result, in 1976, the growth rate of health care expenditures decreased significantly.

Figure 1. **Ambulatory medical care delivery under social sickness funds**

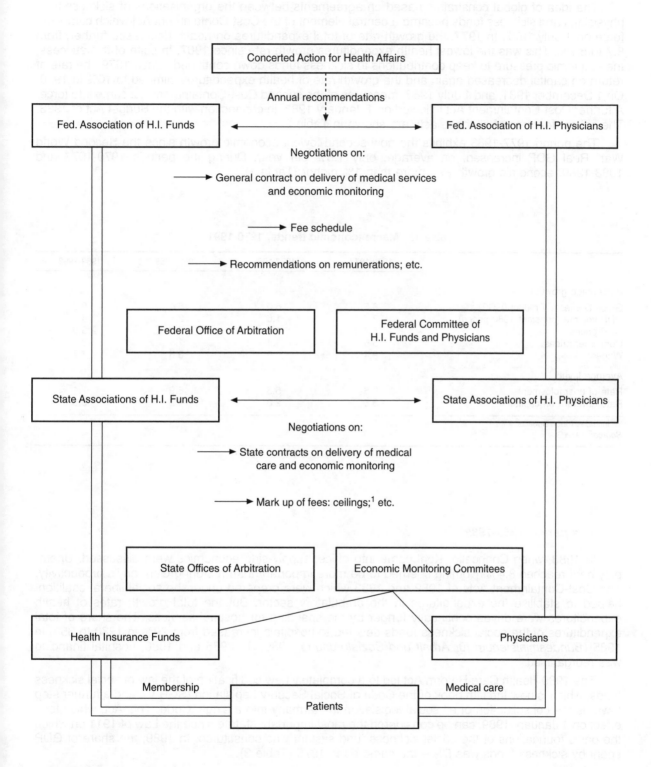

1. Since 1977.

Source: U. Geissler, *Alternative Methods of Physician Compensation and Their Effects on Physician Activity – An International Comparison.* Country Report for the Federal Republic of Germany, CREDOC, Paris 1981, p. 32.

The period 1977-1983

The idea of global constraints based on agreements between the organisations of sickness-fund physicians and sickness funds became a central element of the Cost-Containment Act which came into force on 1 July 1977. In 1977, the growth rate of total expenditures on health decreased further, from 8.7 to 5.7%. This was the lowest health expenditures growth rate since 1967. In spite of this success, the economic pressure to keep contributions to sickness funds down continued. Since 1979, the rate of return on capital decreased again and the growth rate of health expenditures climbed to 10% in 1980. On 1 December 1981, and 1 July 1982, measures of the second Cost-Containment Act came into force. A further Cost-Containment Act followed on 1 January 1983, in connection with the Budget Act of 1983. The salient features of all these acts are shown in Table 2.

The period 1977-1983 exhibits the now second lowest economic growth since the Second World War. Real GDP increased, on average, only 1.6% per year. During the periods 1970-1977 and 1983-1989, economic growth was more than 1% higher (Table 1).

Table 1. **Macroeconomic trends, 1970-1991**

	1970-1977	1977-1983	1983-1989	1989-1992
Percentage growth rates:				
Gross Domestic Product (GDP)	8.5	5.0	5.4	8.2
GDP volume (constant 1980 prices)	2.7	1.6	2.8	4.1
GDP prices	5.7	4.1	2.2	3.9
Consumer prices	5.5	4.4	1.5	3.1
Wages*	9.4	4.5	3.8	7.7
Average level:				
Rate of unemployment	2.6	5.5	8.9	7.1
Rate of return on capital	3.6	2.8	4.2	5.3

*   Includes fringe benefits.
Source: BASYS.

The period 1983-1989

In 1983, when Chancellor Kohl came into office, supply-side economics were discussed. Unemployment reached 8.4%. Nothing seemed to be more important than restoring Germany's productivity. The Cost-Containment Acts of 1982 and 1983 which were prepared under the social-liberal coalition, helped to stabilise the expenditures in the ambulatory sector. But the total growth rates of health expenditures were driven continually further by the spending for hospital services. The share of total expenditures of the social sickness funds devoted to hospitals increased from 29% in 1980 to 35% in 1985 (*Bundesministerium für Arbeit und Sozialordnung,* 1989). In 1985 and 1986, hospital financing was reorganised.

The 1989 Health Care Reform Act led to a completely new codification of the law of social sickness funds, which is now the fifth book of the Code of Social Security Legislation (SGB V), and a further step towards the consolidation of all social legislation in Germany into a single Code. This Act, which took effect on 1 January 1989, can be considered the most important statute since the Law of 1911 on which the basic foundations of the social sickness fund system was constituted. In 1989, the share of GDP spent by sickness funds was 5% – the same as in 1975 (Table 3).

The period since 1989

The fact that hospital expenditures were largely unconsidered in the 1989 Health Care Reform Act proved a major point of criticism. Despite the considerable cost savings in the years 1989 and 1990, the

Table 2. **The Cost-Containment Acts of the Federal Republic of Germany, 1977-1993**

01.07.77   Cost-Containment Act (Krankenversicherungs-Kostendämpfungsgesetz KVKG)

- Creation of the Concerted Action for Health Affairs.
- Coinsurance on prescriptions – 20% of the costs (maximum DM 2.50) – is replaced by a copayment of DM 1 for each drug.
- Cost-reimbursement for dentures is limited to 80%.
- The statutory sickness funds is given the possibility to introduce coinsurance on orthodontics.
- Nursing care at home is obligatory under certain circumstances to reduce in-patient care.
- The costs for home help given by near relatives are no longer reimbursed.
- Family members with income above a certain sum, are no longer free-insured.
- Pensioners are only accepted in social sickness funds if they have been members during their working life.

01.12.81 and 01.07.82   Hospital Cost-Containment Act (Krankenhaus-Kostendämpfungsgesetz)

- Reduction of number of beds is to be accelerated by subsidies.
- Sickness funds must cooperate in the hospital planning of the *Länder*.
- Sickness funds have greater say in determing the level of reimbursement for health care.
- Regulation of hospital care is included in the Concerted Action.

01.12.81 and 01.07.82   Supplementary Cost-Containment Act (Kostendämpfungs-Ergänzungsgesetz)

- Fees for technical dental services are reduced for 1 year by 5%.
- Reimbursement for dentures is changed: insurance pays 100% for the dentists' services and up to 60% of material and laboratory costs.
- Copayments for medical aids and appliances are introduced.
- For medical aids and appliances, the reimbursement prices are fixed until December 31, 1983.
- The copayment on drugs is raised to DM 1.50, and for physiotherapy and glasses to DM 4.
- New glasses are only reimbursable once every 3 years if visual acuity does not change.
- Thermal cures are only granted once every 3 years.
- Handicapped persons can become voluntary members of the social sickness funds if they, or their relatives have been members at least 3 of the preceding 5 years.
- The ALOS after in-patient admission for childbirth is regularly limited to 6 (formerly 10) days.
- A copayment of DM 5 is introduced for transportation costs.

01.01.83   Amended Budget Act (Haushaltsbegleitgesetz 1983)

- Insured persons must pay DM 5 per day (for a maximum 14 days) for in-patient care.
- The copayment on drugs is raised to DM 2 per item.
- Expenses for home help services may be reimbursable, if necessary, to minimize in-patient care.
- Medicines for minor ailments are no longer covered as of April 1, 1983.

01.01.84   Amended Budget Act 1984 (Haushaltsbegleitgesetz 1984)

- Contributions to social sickness funds must be applied on special wages, such as bonuses, tips, etc.
- Patients with sick benefits have to pay contributions to old-age and unemployment insurance; contributions are split between patients and sickness funds.

01.01.85   Hospital Financing Act (Gesetz zur Neuordnung der Krankenhausfinanzierung)

- The present mixed-financing of construction by the Federalal Government and the *Länder* will be shifted to the *Länder*.
- Sickness funds and hospitals may finance certain kinds of investments by per diem rates.

01.01.86   Federal Hospital Payment Regulation (Bundespflegesatzverordnung BPflV)

- The concept of prospective budgets that are agreed upon by sickness funds and hospitals is introduced.
- If the funds and hospitals do not agree, an arbitration board decides.
- It is possible to arrange special daily rates for departments, and special payments for expensive care, *e.g.*, heart operations.
- Funds may inform patients in detail about the care they receive.

01.01.89   Health Care Reform Act (Gesundheits-Reformgesetz GRG)

- Provides choice of type of insurance for blue collar workers with incomes above the assessment ceiling, making the legislation for these workers equal to that already applicable to white collar workers.
- Sickness fund coverage for students is restricted.
- Compulsory insurance is extended to young adults in secondary education programs.
- Compulsory insurance for certain categories of self-employed people is abolished.
- Requirements concerning prior insurance periods for pensioners are tightened.
- Qualifying conditions for voluntary membership in social sickness funds are made stricter.
- Provisions are repealed under which pensioners, civil servants, and self-employed persons could previously enter the scheme.
- Family assistance is established as an autonomous insurance right.
- Coverage of preventive care, *e.g.*, preventive dental care, health check-ups, is extended.
- Concept of "patient pays first, then is reimbursed" is introduced for dentures; coinsurance for dentures is increased from 20 to 50% bonuses are payable if teeth are regularly attended to.
- Reference prices for pharmaceutical products and appliances are introduced.
- Provision of home care is expanded.
- Special services that require continous attendance are made available.

- Certain provisions concerning death benefits are repealed, and certain transitional provisions are made.
- Severe restrictions are placed on reimbursement of travel and transport costs.
- Individual social sickness funds are authorized to introduce new services temporarily on an experimental basis and to test them in pilot conditions.
- In all contracts, the principle of stability of contribution rates should be considered.
- Monitoring medical services is to be conducted on a sample basis.
- Sickness funds may terminate contracts with inefficient hospitals.
- General monitoring is to be done of costs and quality in hospitals; needs for major medical technologies are to be coordinated.
- The minimum contribution payable by voluntarily insured persons is doubled.
- Introduction of compulsory and optional contribution sharing arrangements.

01.01.93 Health Care Structure Act (Gesundheits-Strukturgesetz GStG)

- Insured members of sickness funds get smart cards.
- Total payments of sickness funds for ambulatory services by physicians, for dental care are capped on basis of the payments of the year 1991 and of the increase of the incomes of sickness funds members in the following years; only preventive services are excluded from the budget.
- Payments for ambulatory services of physicians will be cut if prescription volume exceeds a ceilings (malus-regulation).
- The conversion factor for dentures will be diminished 20%.
- Reference prices for material and laboratory services of technical dental services are introduced.
- Discrimination of fees for medical and dental services among groups of sickness fund members, *e.g.*, members of substitute funds and local funds, is abolished.
- Total payments of sickness funds for drugs are capped on the basis of 1991 payments, the growth of sickness fund members, and the growth of drug prices.
- Prices of drugs outside of the reference price system are diminished 5% for the years 1993 and 1994; the pharmaceutical industry is invited to voluntary renounce raising prices of drugs within the reference price system.
- Sickness funds are obliged to inform patients on low-priced medical aids.
- Payments of sickness funds for hospital care are capped on the basis of the 1991 payments. The budgets of the hospitals for the the years 1993, 1994, and 1995 must not exceed the growth of the incomes of sickness fund members.
- The hospital cost-price-reimbursement principle is replaced by reimbursement according to delivered services.
- Financing private hospital investments is improved.
- Sickness funds given the possibility to become shareholders of private non-profit insurance companies due to provide complementary insurance for dentures.
- Sickness funds have to extend monitoring of efficiency and appropriateness of medical services, prescriptions, and hospital admissions.

Source: BASYS (Beratungsgesellschaft für angewandte Systemforschung mbH).

sickness funds again ran into deficits in the years 1991 and 1992. Thus, the Act ended only provisionally the series of cost-containment measures started in 1977 (Table 2). In July 1992, the Ministry of Health submitted the Health Care Structure Act, to be implemented as from January 1993.

Objects of cost-containment acts

With the Cost-Containment Act of 1 July 1977, began a series of Cost-Containment Acts that shared the goal of bringing the development of health care expenditures into line with the growth of wages and salaries of the sickness-fund members. These acts implemented a macro-economic approach of expenditure regulation that has been first and foremost revenue-oriented. That is, the growth of sickness-fund expenditures has been related to the growth of their revenues (contributions based on wages).

A further goal of all Cost-Containment Acts was to preserve free access, independent of income. The limitation of expenditure growth should not result in a limitation of necessary services to the patient. The benefits already granted should, in general, not be reduced. On the contrary, medical progress should be made available to the insured. All members of the social sickness funds should have access to high standards of medical care. The crucial point of Cost-Containment Acts, however, is the fact that (with very few exceptions) services have not been limited. Members of the sickness funds have unlimited access to a complete range of medical and dental care.

The challenge of cost containment was not only to avoid negative effects on medical progress and access to medical care, but also to give sickness funds effective measures to stabilise their financial situation which requires high contributions because of the low wages of their members. It is necessary to keep in mind that the contribution rates of the members of the 1 123 social sickness funds vary greatly. The contribution base consists mainly of wages, salaries and pensions. Thus the contributions are completely independent of individual risks of medical treatment costs. In January 1992, the average contribution rate was 12.46%. This means that an industrial worker with an average gross monthly income of DM 3 700 paid DM 461 in monthly contributions. But the variations of individuals' ability to pay, and in the health risks of the members, have led to great variations in the fund's contribution rates. On 1 January 1992, the contribution rates for both employer and employee ranged from 8 to 16.5%. So the maximum contribution was DM 841.50 per month for an industrial worker with a monthly income equal to the income ceiling of DM 5 100.

To achieve the goal of income-orientated expenditure growth, the increase of expenditures on certain kinds of care was tied to the increase in the so-called *Grundlohnsumme,* that is the income of the sickness-funds members. In other words, the expenditure increase was linked to the average insurable wage on which the contribution to the sickness-fund system is calculated. The point has been made that the linkage between expenditures for health and economic data does not fully correspond to the needs for health services. The marginal increase of the *Grundlohnsumme* is actually the result of the bargaining between employers and labour unions, and does not reflect the marginal increase in needs.

To limit the increase in sickness-fund expenditures, recommendations were introduced at the federal level to contain the growth rates of the total payments to both physicians and hospitals. These recommendations were addressed to the negotiations between physicians and sickness funds at the state level, because it is at this level that overall sickness-fund payments to physicians are set. In determining the rate of increase of the expenditure cap for payments to physicians, several factors have to be taken into consideration, including the increase in workers' annual income, office costs, physician working time, and the expansion of services justified by epidemics or progress in medical research.

The Cost-Containment Act of 1977 created an on-going programme at the federal level called Concerted Action for Health Affairs (CAHA). Its purpose is to discuss and agree upon recommendations concerning the growth rates of spending for ambulatory medical care, dental care, and drugs. Additionally, CAHA deals with major problems connected with the provision of medical care. Participants develop recommendations to improve efficacy and increase efficiency in health care. On the basis of the findings of CAHA, providers and funds negotiate their contracts. The CAHA meets twice a year. Meetings are prepared by a committee composed of members of the Concerted Action. In every year's first meeting (which takes place before 31 March), the recommendations concerning the increase of the global compensations for physicians and dentists, and the global sum to be spent on prescriptions have to be voted upon. In the second meeting, which takes place in the autumn, matters concerning the effectiveness, efficiency, and the rationalisation of the health care system are discussed as well as matters concerning the development of medical and economic background data to guide policy.

CAHA has 64 members, including physicians, pharmacists and dentists as well as representatives of the sickness funds, private health insurance companies, hospitals, the pharmaceutical industry, trade unions, and employers. The *Länder,* the counties and the municipalities are also represented in this conference. CAHA is convened by the Federal Ministry of Health (formerly the Ministry of Labour and Social Affairs). This Ministry is now responsible for the social sickness funds. Other federal ministries are represented but cannot vote.

The Cost-Containment Act of 1977 also introduced regulations intended to reduce costs. These regulations relate to the provision of home help and home nursing care, the restriction of rest and recuperation in spas, the connection between ambulatory and in-patient care, and user charges.

When efforts to restrain expenditure growth were beginning, CAHA discussed the idea of cost containment in hospitals but without the right to make recommendations. As a result, there were complaints from the physicians, dentists, pharmacists, the pharmaceutical industry, and the sickness funds that the hospitals, which caused the highest share of expenditures for the sickness funds, were not bound by recommendations concerning increase of expenditures. This situation was changed by the act of 1982. This second Cost-Containment Act also increased user charges for drugs and physiotherapy.

Since 1986, in its annual reports, a board of seven advisers to the CAHA provides medical and economic guidelines to serve as a basis for recommendations.

The Health Care Reform Act (HCRA) of 1989 was not designed to be a radical revision of the current system of health insurance. Services and benefits covered by the "principle of solidarity" should be redesigned. The principle of solidarity requires equal financial burdens in financing services for major health care needs. To avoid negative effects caused by "free riders" and high contribution rates, only medically necessary services should be included in the health care baskets of the sickness funds. Further objectives of the HCRA were to encourage individuals to take greater responsibility for their life style, and for using services as sparingly as possible. HCRA also strengthened the role of sickness funds' administrations to enable them to monitor the efficiency of physicians and hospitals, and to contract out any "bad apples".

Although the HCRA of 1989 amended the law of the social sickness funds completely, a need for further reforms has been demanded towards risks. Inequality of treatment of blue- and white-collar employees regarding choice of sickness fund still exists. Thus, an organisational reform has been announced to the current legislature which started in 1991. But the economic pressure to finance the reunification process and the reconstruction of the economic system in the Eastern states of Germany, the sluggish pace of economic growth as well as the rising deficits of sickness funds since 1991, changed the priorities of reforms. The objective of the Health Care Structure Act (HCSA) of 1993 is, again, cost containment. The expenditures of all major functions of the health care system are to be capped to avoid increases of contribution rates.

Supply effects

Any regular supply curve slopes upward, indicating that the higher the price, the greater the amount offered. A lower price leads to lower production. It is obvious that this traditional view of the supply curve indicates a contradiction between the goals of Cost-Containment Acts to reduce expenditures without limiting access to medical services.

In fact, there was much criticism of health care providers concerning the overall CAHA recommendations and their effects on quality of medical care. Compared with other professions, physicians' and dentists' real incomes have decreased since 1980. One must question how far the income level can be reduced without jeopardising the economic situation of physicians and dentists working in out-patient practices. The question arises as to how overall recommendations on the yearly increase of expenditures can be put into practice in a situation where some 100 000 physicians and dentists practice privately. Also, how can a recommendation on the increase of expenditures on drugs be put into effect in a situation where some 1 000 pharmaceutical firms work in a free market system? Further, how could increases in spending for medical progress, *e.g.* research and development of new drugs, be held to fixed growth rates?

Office-based physicians

Ambulatory medical services are provided by office-based doctors. More than 80% of their revenue come from sickness funds: all reimbursement activities of the sickness funds directly affect the incomes of the doctors.

Both social and private sickness funds pay for ambulatory medical services on a fee-for-service basis. The current fee schedule for physicians' services supplied to members of the social sickness funds was established in 1978. Since then, the structure of the schedule as well as the fees for the various services have been changed as a result of the negotiations between the national and regional organisations of the different sickness funds and the organisations of sickness-fund physicians. In general, physician reimbursement for a given service differs because, traditionally, the white-collar workers' funds pay higher fees. Physicians are reimbursed on the basis of a legal fee schedule containing even higher rates for services supplied to people with private insurance. The differences in physician pay led to a system of multiple standards, which is occasionally reflected in differing waiting times and differing face-to-face contact with the physicians.

The measures of cost containment on ambulatory medical care have been primarily price-containment measures. While, on the average, expenditures for ambulatory medical care grew at an annual rate of 5.9% between 1977 and 1991, fees increased at a mere 1.3% annual rate (BASYS and CREDES, 1992).

In spite of the cost containment, the number of office-based physicians increased by more than 2% annually since 1977 (Table 3). By the end of 1991, their number reached 77 541. That is, 21 384 or 28% more than in 1977 (Kassenärztliche Bundesvereinigung, 1992). Therefore, the revenue per physician

Table 3. **Share of health expenditure funding in gross domestic product, 1970-1992**

(in percentage)

	Total	Social sickness funds	Old-age and accident insurance	Federal *Länder* local authorities	Private health insurance	Other
1970	5.35	3.00	0.35	0.73	0.44	0.83
1971	5.85	3.37	0.36	0.84	0.44	0.83
1972	6.14	3.61	0.38	0.88	0.44	0.83
1973	6.48	3.88	0.39	0.94	0.43	0.84
1974	7.12	4.39	0.43	0.96	0.48	0.86
1975	7.83	5.02	0.42	0.99	0.50	0.89
1976	7.80	5.08	0.38	0.95	0.50	0.88
1977	7.72	5.00	0.37	0.96	0.49	0.91
1978	7.76	5.00	0.36	1.02	0.50	0.89
1979	7.66	4.98	0.36	0.93	0.51	0.87
1980	7.94	5.17	0.38	0.95	0.53	0.91
1981	8.26	5.36	0.39	1.02	0.57	0.92
1982	8.17	5.24	0.38	1.01	0.58	0.96
1983	8.06	5.18	0.33	0.97	0.56	1.02
1984	8.20	5.33	0.32	0.94	0.56	1.04
1985	8.35	5.39	0.33	0.99	0.57	1.07
1986	8.26	5.37	0.33	0.96	0.57	1.04
1987	8.33	5.41	0.34	0.95	0.59	1.03
1988	8.57	5.57	0.34	0.96	0.60	1.10
1989	8.17	5.06	0.34	0.97	0.62	1.17
1990	8.15	5.07	0.33	0.97	0.63	1.14
1991	8.27	5.20	0.33	0.96	0.66	1.12
1992*						

* The 1992 estimates are preliminary.
Source: BASYS.

increased more slowly than the total increase of expenditures for physicians' services. Whereas total population remained virtually the same since 1977, the number of patients per office decreased steadily.

The supply side has reacted price containment by increasing the quantity of services per patient. This holds especially true for those services with low marginal costs, like laboratory tests. But because the total of revenues are fixed by the sickness funds, more services did not automatically lead to more revenues per physician. On the contrary, more services are outweighed by price drops as the average conversion factor of fees decreases due to the reimbursement ceiling and the increase in the number of physicians. As yet, there has been no fundamental reaction on the part of the supply side to this increased economic pressure. Obviously, the incomes of office-based physicians seem to be high enough to bear such a cost-containment policy.

Dentists

In Germany, per capita expenditures for dental care are the highest in the world (Schneider *et al.,* 1990). This is mainly because of high expenditures for dentures which have been nearly fully covered by sickness funds since 1974. Table 5 shows annual growth rates of 18.8% during the period 1970-1977, before cost containment. In this period the number of practising dentists was relatively stable at some 27 000 (Kassenzahnärztliche Bundesvereinigung, 1990). Increased demand did not affect this number until 1980. Since 1980, however, the number of practising dentists is growing by 2% annually (Table 4). This growth rate is higher than that for utilisation of dental care, which shows the lowest growth of all health care services in the 1980s (Table 6).

For members of the sickness funds, dentists bill are based on the common fee schedule for dental services. Claims of dentists are settled similarly to the way those of physicians are – through *Land* dentist organisations, which in turn settle up quarterly with the sickness funds. For dentures, the HCRA of 1989 changed the payment method, so dentists now have to bill the patient directly; sickness funds then reimburse patients.

Table 4. Increase in medical and para-medical care providers, 1970-1991

(average annual rate of increase, in percentage)

	1970-1977	1977-1991
Active physicians	3.9	3.5
Office-based physicians	1.7	2.3
Hospital physicians	7.1	3.9
Active dentists	−0.1	1.6
Pharmacists	3.7	2.4
Hospital beds	0.8	−0.7
Hospital staff	3.8	1.8
Nurses	5.6	4.4

Source: BASYS.

Table 5. Health expenditure by functions, 1970-1992

(in millions DM)

	Total[1]	Physician services[2]	Dental services	Pharmaceutical goods	Hospital services	Others[3]
1970	36 117	7 327	3 946	7 124	12 014	5 687
1971	43 852	9 156	4 884	8 142	14 854	6 817
1972	50 587	10 313	5 652	9 176	17 426	8 020
1973	59 493	11 660	6 666	10 431	21 123	9 613
1974	70 048	13 519	8 004	11 956	25 302	11 267
1975	80 374	14 624	11 035	13 226	28 578	12 911
1976	87 384	15 516	12 528	14 094	30 337	14 909
1977	92 345	16 261	13 234	14 547	32 252	16 051
1978	99 639	17 298	14 302	15 743	34 551	17 744
1979	106 334	18 652	15 741	16 753	36 364	18 824
1980	116 920	20 207	17 424	18 536	40 082	20 671
1981	126 842	21 879	19 084	19 851	43 517	22 511
1982	129 776	22 530	7 898	20 792	45 287	23 269
1983	134 570	23 370	17 738	22 010	46 724	24 728
1984	143 574	24 642	18 975	23 323	49 558	27 076
1985	152 231	25 706	19 631	24 938	52 912	29 044
1986	159 111	26 624	19 555	25 992	55 771	31 171
1987	166 288	27 798	19 017	27 508	58 182	33 783
1988	180 202	28 964	24 015	29 566	60 946	36 790
1989	181 740	30 649	21 046	29 891	62 601	37 522
1990	195 352	33 100	21 915	31 984	68 524	39 830
1991	213 544	36 131	24 620	35 182	74 877	42 733
1992[4]						

Average annual growth in nominal prices (in percentage)						
1970-1977	14.4	12.1	18.8	10.7	15.2	16.0
1977-1992[4]	6.2	5.9	4.6	6.5	6.2	7.5

1. Health expenditure as defined here does not include cash benefits, administration, construction, research and development.
2. Ambulatory care only.
3. Includes medical aids and appliances, long-term care and other services.
4. The 1992 estimates and 1977-1992 growth rates are preliminary.
Source: BASYS.

Although there was no cap comparable to that for ambulatory medical services during most years of cost containment, the actual growth rates of expenditures for dental care (excluding dentures) have been lower than the CAHA-recommended levels (Berg, 1986). One explanation for this development has been the relative values of fees in the common fee schedule. Restorations were undervalued, crowns and dentures overvalued. This distortion in the relative values of the fee schedule encouraged dentists to provide crowns and dentures. In 1986, the common fee schedule for dental services was

Table 6. **Real health expenditures growth, 1970-1992**

(percentage)

	Total[1]	Physician services[2]	Dental services	Pharmaceutical goods	Hospital services[3]
1971	9.7	8.4	16.9	9.0	4.5
1972	8.4	6.6	13.1	8.2	2.5
1973	9.7	7.3	13.5	8.9	3.2
1974	8.7	7.5	11.1	9.7	4.2
1975	8.6	5.4	26.9	5.8	0.5
1976	5.3	3.0	9.2	4.6	1.2
1977	2.1	0.7	2.9	0.3	2.4
1978	4.8	4.8	5.3	5.9	2.0
1979	2.5	4.5	5.9	2.4	0.1
1980	4.5	5.5	7.4	5.2	2.0
1981	2.6	3.9	4.5	4.0	-0.5
1982	0.0	3.2	-7.5	0.8	0.2
1983	1.2	2.8	-2.5	1.7	0.1
1984	4.3	3.6	4.9	3.3	3.4
1985	3.6	2.4	2.4	3.8	4.0
1986	3.6	3.7	-2.0	3.6	4.2
1987	3.6	6.9	-4.8	5.0	0.9
1988	8.4	10.7	18.9	5.5	4.1
1989	-0.7	1.4	-9.7	-0.3	1.5
1990	4.5	4.1	1.1	5.5	3.7
1991	5.6	5.6	9.3	8.1	3.5
1992[4]					
			Average annual growth		
1970-1977	7.5	5.5	13.2	6.6	2.6
1977-1992[4]	3.4	4.5	2.0	3.8	2.1

1. Health expenditure as defined here does not include cash benefits, administration, construction, research and development.
2. Ambulatory care only.
3. Excludes a number of long-term institutions.
4. The 1992 estimates and 1977-1992 growth rates are preliminary.
Source: BASYS.

completely revised. Further, since 1 July 1986, special guidelines came into force to ensure the use of cost-effective material for dentures. Price containment of dental care is also a central issue of the Health Care Structure Act of 1993, which provides reference prices for the materials used to prepare dentures, as well as an overall reduction of fees for dentures.

Pharmaceuticals

The Cost-Containment Act of 1977 required that the federal organisation of sickness-fund physicians and the federal associations of the sickness funds recommend a maximum budget for prescriptions. If the maximum was exceeded, steps had to be taken to identify what caused the overrun. If the excess expenditures did not arise from an unpredictable increase in morbidity, there were no mechanisms to keep the increase within the budget. Therefore, it was not surprising that the annual growth rates of pharmaceutical expenditures were only one year behind those recommended by CAHA. However, after the Cost-Containment Act of 1977, the real growth rates of pharmaceutical expenditures were reduced to one-half the previous amount.

The *Land* exerts no influence with respect to drug price-fixing at the production level. Pharmaceutical products are priced according to the prevailing market situation. The cost of production, the quality and price of competing products, the prescription habits of physicians, the regulations required by the federal government regarding safety, efficacy and price are among the factors that influence the price decisions of each pharmaceutical firm. The pharmacist's selling price is based on the wholesale mark-up and the pharmacist's own mark-up, the limits of both being defined by law.

Although the real growth of expenditures for drugs during the period 1977-1991 may have been reduced by nearly one-half to that of the span before cost containment (Table 6), the share spent for drugs was rather high. This was because of high prescription rates and high prices. In comparison to other member States of the European Community, Germany has very high drug prices (Sermeus and Adriaenssens, 1989).

In recent years, the government has introduced measures to enforce price competition in the pharmaceutical market. The parliament created a so-called Revision Commission, the task of which is to publish and distribute lists comparing prices and medical compounds having the same uses and/or ingredients.

There are also several lists available to physicians in which information is available on price, composition, quality, etc. These lists are published by the pharmaceutical industry, by researchers, and by the Revision Commission. Further price-containment measures have included the monitoring of physician prescribing habits and voluntary price containment by the pharmaceutical industry. In spite of these activities, during the period 1983-1989, prescription prices increased more than consumer prices (Tables 1 and 7).

With the HCRA of 1989, the reimbursement policy of the sickness funds changed significantly. For drugs with suitable substitutes, reimbursement is set at the price level of generics. Insured people are given incentives to use cheaper medicines, without restricting their entitlement to medically sound pharmaceutical products in any way. In addition, competition among manufacturers of pharmaceutical products should be promoted. From the standpoint of the insured, the reference price system will operate as follows: sickness funds will pay the full cost of any generic medicine for which a reference price has been established. If the insured person uses a more expensive medicine, he or she pays the amount in excess of the reference price. For medicines for which no reference price has been set, there is a co-payment of DM 3 per item.

According to the HCRA of 1989, reference prices are planned for the following types of medicines:
- Drugs with the same active ingredients.
- Drugs with pharmacologically comparable active ingredients, especially chemically related ingredients.
- Drugs with comparable pharmacological-therapeutic effect, in particular drug combinations.

The allocation of medicines to these groups must take into account that the range of possibilities of treatment is not thereby reduced, and that medically sound prescription alternatives are available. Reference prices are fixed jointly by the federal organisations of sickness funds and physicians. These organisations must ensure an adequate supply of effective medicines of guaranteed quality at reasonable prices. The amounts set are to be reviewed regularly and adjusted in light of changes in the market situation. The overall savings of the reference price system are anticipated to reach approximately DM 2 billion yearly.

The first steps in the introduction of the reference price system have already been made. The first reference prices were set, on average, at 30% below the previous prices of the brand name products (Schwabe and Paffrath, 1990). Subsequently pharmaceutical companies reduced their prices to the levels of the reference system. In December 1989, prices of drugs with fixed rates dropped by 21%, whereas the prices of drugs without fixed rates rose by 2.1%.

The HCRA of 1989 also promoted drug substitution. On the prescription form, the doctor is *obliged* to specify whether the pharmacist is allowed to dispense a cheaper generic. Since 1981, the percentage of generics prescriptions has gone up from 7.2 to 21.9% (Schwabe and Paffrath, 1990).

Hospitals

The Hospital Law of 1972 had considerable influence on the expenditures of the social sickness funds. Until then, the hospital owners had the responsibility for the construction of hospitals – public, private, or voluntary – subsidised by *Land* funds. The amount of subsidies was determined by each Land, and showed considerable variation. The daily hospital rate was the result of negotiations between the hospital and the sickness funds. The rate never covered actual costs, and the hospital had to make up the deficit.

With the Hospital Law of 1972, the construction of hospitals became a matter of public interest. The daily charge was fixed by the hospitals, the sickness funds, and the *Länder* at the beginning of the planning period (for one year), and had to cover the expected current or operating costs of the hospital, including the salaries for hospital physicians. The *Länder* were required to develop plans for the number and distribution of hospital beds. Construction and restoration of hospitals were subsidised up to 100% from public funds according to the hospital plan (Beske, 1982).

The Law led to the construction of a considerable number of modern hospitals containing a greater number of beds with up-to-date major equipment. During the period 1970-1977, hospital services showed the highest percentage rise of prices when compared with other services (Table 7).

Cost containment of hospital expenditures was never effectively included in CAHA. The major obstacles have been the dual financing of current services and construction. Nevertheless, the recommendations of CAHA have influenced the growth rates of daily charges. In connection with the guidelines for hospital staff per bed, the annual growth rate of hospital prices was reduced to 4.0% for the period 1989-1991 compared with 12.2% for the period 1970-1977 (Table 7).

The Hospital Financing Act and the Federal Hospital Payment Regulation – which came into existence in 1985 and 1986, respectively – implemented a prospective budget system that allows for profits in a certain range. The prospective budget includes all operating costs (*i.e.* staff and resources costs). Investment costs are included only to a very small extent, as they are predominantly financed via public *Land* subsidies. All hospitals have to set up a standard cost and service record, providing an overview of their cost structure. The Hospital Financing Act also contains several alternative payment forms. Besides the basic daily rate, special compensation rates may be introduced. It is proposed to develop a uniform federal special compensation scheme with aproximately 100 to 120 compensation rates.

Although the ratio of hospital beds per 1 000 population has decreased from 1.18 in 1977 to 1.09 in 1988 (BASYS and CREDES, 1990) it is notable that, despite this reduction, Germany has the highest density of acute care beds in the European Community. There is a wide range in the scale of hospital beds per 1 000 population among German *Länder,* with 9.5 at the bottom of the range and 15.4 at the top (Statistisches Bundesamt, 1989). Some of these differences can, of course, be explained by the proportion of elderly, and the existence of medical teaching faculties in urban versus rural areas. On the other hand, such a wide range indicates that there is an excessive supply of acute care beds in some

Table 7. **Nominal and real growth of health expenditures, 1970-1992**

(average annual rates in percentage)

	1970-1977	1977-1983	1983-1989	1989-1991
Nominal prices (value):				
Total[1]	14.4	6.5	5.1	5.8
Physician services[2]	12.1	6.2	4.6	5.4
Pharmaceuticals	10.7	7.2	5.2	6.2
Dental services	18.8	5.0	2.9	4.1
Hospital services[3]	15.2	6.4	4.9	5.7
Constant 1980 prices (volume):				
Total[1]	7.5	2.6	3.7	5.1
Physician services[2]	5.5	4.1	4.4	5.3
Pharmaceuticals	6.6	3.3	3.3	6.8
Dental services	13.2	2.0	0.9	5.1
Hospital services[3]	2.6	0.6	3.0	3.6
Prices:				
Total[1]	6.4	3.8	1.3	2.7
Physician services[2]	6.2	2.0	–0.1	1.3
Pharmaceuticals	3.9	3.7	1.9	2.6
Dental services	5.0	2.9	2.0	2.5
Hospital services[3]	12.2	5.7	1.9	4.0

1. Health expenditure as defined here does not include cash benefits, administration, construction, research and development.
2. Ambulatory care only.
3. Does not include all long-term care institutions.
Source: BASYS.

areas, a view supported by the fact that German *Länder* with fewer acute care beds do not complain about hospital deficiencies.

The pressure to contain daily charges has helped, indeed, to reduce the expansion of hospital costs, but it has also delayed the adjustment of the hospital capacities to become more efficient. In Germany, the average length of stay (ALOS) and the bed density are higher, and the staff per bed is lower than in other Western countries.

Demand effects

As pointed out, cost-containment policy has been primarily price-containment policy. Containment of utilisation was designed to play only a supplementary role. The following measures were introduced as part of the cost-containment legislation to limit the quantity of services delivered:

- Reduction in entitlement to benefits.
- Reimbursement limits per case, combined with monitoring.
- User charges.

Most health politicians and administrators in Germany believe that co-insurance or co-payment regulations are ineffective and have negative distributional effects. People should have free access to medical services. The physician carries the responsibility for avoiding unnecessary services. Therefore, user charges are not the appropriate measure to reduce supplier-induced demand, if such exists.

Despite these orientations, since the enactment of the Cost-Containment Act of 1977, user charges have been revised several times and increased in certain health services. Various exemptions have been introduced to take care of indigents. At present, children and teenagers under 18 years are exempt from co-insurance, except for dentures and transport costs. An exemption from co-insurance is also possible if medical goods with reference prices (*e.g.*, drugs or glasses) are involved. Also exempted are persons collecting unemployment and those enrolled in higher education. Furthermore, there are limits to co-insurance in accordance with the income of the insured.

Altogether, real expenditures (in 1980 prices) increased during the period 1970-1991 from DM 63 billion to almost DM 167 billion. Compared with 1977, the major effect of cost containment on demand was on dental care, which increased, on average, only 2.0% annually, followed by hospital care, with 2.1% annually (in 1980 prices). Since 1977, the highest increase in demand is for ambulatory care by physicians, to date, which is the only function without user charges (Table 7).

Ambulatory physician services

Patients are free to choose any doctor. However, since 1984, patients covered by sickness funds may claim only one treatment voucher per quarter. (The patient submits the voucher to the physician at the beginning of a treatment. The physician lists his services for all visits by the patient during the quarter on the backside of the voucher.) Patients must obtain a referral certificate for visits to any other doctor. In practice, this restriction is of minor importance. Analyses of treatment vouchers in particular exhibit a rise in the referral certificates and services delivered per voucher.

Because of the existing agreements of remuneration, an increase in vouchers and in the quantity of services per voucher does not result in a proportionate increase in the total remuneration. Nevertheless, physicians compete with each other, and therefore, the individual physician is interested in increasing services to maintain his income.

Although patients of sickness funds do not face user charges for office visits, the figures indicate demand effects of the HCRA of 1989. Real expenditures increased by 10.7% in 1988 and dropped to an increase of 1.4% in 1989 (Table 6). This reaction of demand may be partly explained by patient uncertainty concerning actual user charges, and by increase in user charges for prescriptions.

Dental services

In 1974, in the pre-cost-containment period, the demand for dental care was stimulated by a decision of the Supreme Court of Social Affairs, which held that insured people should be covered for dentures in case of missing teeth. In 1975, the real expenditures for dental care increased by 26.9%.

The introduction of a co-insurance rate of 20% for dentures with the Cost-Containment Act of 1977 reduced the demand temporarily (Table 6).

The announcement of the HCRA of 1989 led to anticipatory effects in 1988. In the area of dentures (where user charges increased from about 20 to 50%), the number of cases paid for through the organisation of sickness-funds dentists rose by 21%. Expenditures for dentures increased by 27%. It is worth noting in this context that expenditures for dentures decreased in 1986 (–10.0%) and in 1987 (–8.9%) because of reductions of fees in the common fee schedule. In 1989, when higher user charges came into force, expenditures for dentures dropped by 46%.

Despite the co-insurance rate of 50%, the expenditures for dentures of sickness-fund patients increased by 16% in 1991. Therefore, the cost-containment measures of the 1993 HCSA anticipate a 20% reduction of the conversion factor for dentures. Additionally, reference prices for material and laboratory services of technical dental services are being introduced.

Pharmaceuticals

The first Cost-Containment Act of 1977 introduced a co-payment of DM 1 per prescription. In 1982 the charge had been inflated to DM 1.50 and in 1983 to DM 2. Since 1989, the insured faces a co-payment of DM 3 for a prescribed drug which has, as yet, no reference price. Since 1 June 1989, for drugs with reference prices, the patient has had to pay the difference between the reference price and the actual retail price. For drugs without a reference, the rate of DM 3 will remain until the end of 1991. From 1 July 1993, a coinsurance equal to 15% of the price of the drug with a maximum of DM 10 per item will be required.

All these changes in user charges had significant effects on demand, even if the changes were temporary. In addition, cost-containment acts have tried to control demand through improved monitoring of prescribing behaviour of physicians and through "negative lists". These are lists of items that are not reimbursable for patients 18 years of age or over. Prescribed drugs in the following areas are on negative lists:

- Drugs for colds and flu-type infections including decongestants, analgesics, antitussives and expectorants.
- Any medicines for the mouth or throat, excluding fungal infections.
- Laxatives.
- Travel sickness remedies.

More than two-thirds of the turnover of pharmacies are reimbursed directly by the social sickness funds. Consequently, all measures of the social sickness funds concerning the reimbursement for prescribed medicines are very important for the pharmaceutical market in the Germany.

Hospital services

Patients are essentially free to choose any hospital, although all admissions to a hospital are strictly by referral. According to the HCRA of 1 January 1989, the doctor making the referral must take into account the cost-effectiveness of the hospital in question. A comparative price list of hospitals is currently being compiled. As long as the prices of hospitals are not comparable, this price list may have only minor effects.

From January 1983 through December 1990, patients had to pay DM 5 for each calendar day in a hospital from the first day of admission and for a maximum of 14 days within any calendar year. This co-payment was increased to DM 10 on 1 January 1991. The co-payment is forwarded to the sickness funds. Patients treated in spa clinics or rehabilitation clinics pay DM 15 per day to the sickness funds (with exemptions for indigents and special cases). This does not apply to children up to the age of 18, nor to any period of partial hospitalisation.

It is questionable whether the low co-payment has even a negligible effect on demand for hospital services. However, hospital days per capita reached its lowest point during the period 1977-1988 with 3.37 days. Although the ALOS fell from 20.8 days in 1977 to 16.6 days in 1988, utilisation of hospitals remained quite stable. Average bed days per capita were 3.56 in 1977 and 3.46 in 1988 (BASYS and CREDES, 1990). One reason for the relatively long ALOS and the high use of hospital services in Germany is the way in which ambulatory care and hospital care are kept separate. Therefore, HCRA of

1989 introduced measures to improve the division of labour in both functions. Patients referred to hospital who are not confined to bed should, under certain circumstances (for example before or after an operation) be treated on an out-patient basis. This should either reduce or avoid the need for some hospital admissions.

Structural effects

Public/private mix of care

All cost-containment measures in the sickness fund system have influenced directly or indirectly the private sector. The main cause of this influence is the public assistance for civil servants, almost all of whom are privately insured. Therefore, several cost-containment measures directed to sickness fund expenditures (such as user charges) are usually made applicable for civil servants. On the other hand, payment systems of the private sector differ from those of the public sector.

The principle of patient indemnisation applies to private patients in the area of ambulatory care, *i.e.*, they pay the full cost of any bill to the provider, and are subsequently reimbursed by their health insurance. Civil servants submit their invoices both to the local payment office of their employers, and to their private health insurance plan. The public employers reimburse, in general, 50-70% of the bills, depending on familiy status.

The fee schedule for private patients differs from that for the sickness-fund members. On average, the fees for private medical treatment are twice as high as those of the sickness funds. The private fee schedule was revised in 1965, 1982 and 1988. No studies are available concerning the effects on quality of the higher fees for private services. A study in the Munich area showed that physicians dedicated more time to private patients than to sickness-funds patients (Neubauer and Birkner, 1980). Furthermore, the sickness funds monitor regularly all claims of the physicians. The private health insurance schemes usually monitor only those invoices which exceed a certain threshold.

In contrast to the social sector, the private fee schedule is also applied in hospitals. The hospital physicians (usually senior consultants) bill private patients directly for medical services. On admission, the patient signs a declaration accepting liability for the costs. Then, charges for in-patient care are paid directly to the hospital by the private health insurance companies. Charges are based on the number of care days, and private patients pay an additional charge over and above the per diem set for sickness-fund patients. The daily charge for private patients is, on the one hand, lower than for social patients, because of the direct billing of costs of private medical treatment by hospital physicians. On the other hand, the per diem for private patients covers additional services, such as a private room, that come with private insurance. On average, the total costs per hospital case are about twice as high for private patients as for patients who have social health insurance coverage.

Private spending accounts for less than one-quarter of all health spending in Germany. Since the beginning of cost containment in the mid-1970s, the private share (as well as the number of privately insured people) has increased steadily. The additional demand for nursing care was not covered by the sickness funds, and price inflation of services covered by private insurance has been greater than that for the social funds.

Of importance in this analysis is the validity of the price indexes involved, each developed by using different statistics. The hospital cost-price index is based on per diem costs adjusted to productivity gains by falling ALOS. The public price indexes of ambulatory physician and dental care reflect the rise of point values of the fee schedules. The prices of private physician services are determined by the average fee. This last concept may lead to an overestimation of the price increase of services for patients with private insurance.

In the period 1977-1992, prices for private health care rose annually by 3.5%. During the same time, prices of public health care rose by 2.5% (Table 8). This means that prices for private health care increased more than consumer prices. In contrast, the increase in public prices was below the general inflation rate. This lower increase of public prices was mainly the result of the sickness funds' expenditure cap for ambulatory physician services. This cap steadily reduced the conversion factor of the common fee schedule.

Table 8.   **Private and public mix of health expenditures and its compositional growth, 1970-1992**

(in percentage)

	Private share in total expenditure[1]	Growth rates of:			
		The volume of public expenditure	The prices of public expenditure	The volume of private expenditure	The prices of private expenditure
1970	23.7	–	–	–	–
1971	21.7	11.6	11.6	4.0	7.0
1972	20.8	9.6	6.5	4.6	5.6
1973	19.6	11.2	7.3	4.9	5.8
1974	18.8	9.7	8.4	5.5	7.0
1975	17.8	10.3	5.2	1.9	6.9
1976	17.7	5.7	3.0	2.9	5.3
1977	18.1	1.7	3.5	3.3	4.2
1978	17.9	5.1	2.9	3.0	3.6
1979	18.1	2.2	4.1	4.0	4.3
1980	18.1	4.7	5.1	3.9	5.7
1981	18.0	2.7	5.7	2.1	5.7
1982	18.9	–0.7	2.0	2.9	4.0
1983	19.6	0.7	2.1	3.1	4.3
1984	19.6	4.3	2.3	4.3	2.3
1985	19.7	3.8	2.0	2.4	3.7
1986	19.4	4.0	0.8	2.0	1.3
1987	19.5	4.2	0.3	2.2	2.0
1988	19.9	8.9	–0.9	6.3	3.9
1989	21.9	–2.8	1.3	8.8	2.5
1990	21.8	4.8	3.2	4.5	2.4
1991	21.5	6.0	3.8	5.4	3.1
1992[2]					
Averages					
1970-1977	19.8	8.5	6.5	3.9	6.0
1977-1992[2]	19.5	3.3	2.5	3.5	3.5

1.   Health expenditure as defined here does not include cash benefits, administration, construction, research and development.
2.   The 1992 estimates and 1977-1992 growth rates are preliminary.
Source: BASYS.

Range of contribution rates

During the period 1977-1991, the average contribution rate of the sickness funds – shared equally between the employee and the employer – increased from 11.5 to 12.5% of the employee's income. However, great differences in contribution rates are hidden by these averages. Contribution rates were between 7 and 14.2% as of 1 July 1978; by January 1992 they ranged from 8 to 16.5%. The various Cost-Containment Acts have not reduced the differences among contribution rates. Therefore, the sickness fund system is in need of further reforms. Although the 1989 HCRA amended the Law of the social funds completely, the freedom of choice to subscribe to sickness funds remains unequally available to blue- and white-collar workers. An organisational reform has been announced to establish uniform rules concerning freedom of fund choice and narrower contribution rates.

Wage effect on national income

The relative stability of the share of GDP devoted to health care in the 1980s results partially from the decreasing share of wages in national income. Linking health expenditures to wages can lead to differences between general economic growth and the growth of health care, if wages increase more (or less) than economic growth. During the periods 1976-1979 and 1983-1991, economic growth surpassed the increase in wages. Therefore, the linkage between wages and sickness fund expenditures led to additional profit and interest gains. The linkage to the wage base of contributions enforces the economic cycle, and, as expected, the share of GDP devoted to health care increased as the economic growth was going down in 1991, high inflation pushing the costs of health care.

The Health Care Structure Act of 1993 tries to stop rising shares of GDP devoted to health care by strict budgeting regulations of all major categories of health care and by price containment. The aim is to shift the burden of uncontrolled growth of the utilisation of services to the providers. It is planned to oblige the self-regulation by the associations of funds and organisations of physicians and hospitals to make their contracts of budgets within the limits of the expected wage increase. Starting in 1993, at the outset of each year, the Ministry of Health will announce this expected growth rate.

Future problems

The cost-containment policy of the German health care system has been directed mainly towards reducing price inflation, although the volume of services is a concern in the budgeting of health care costs. This policy has proved useful in keeping down contribution rates and enforcing economic growth. However, in the long run this policy leads to lower quality or to cuts in health care supply as cost inflation surpasses the reimbursement of costs. The federal government has anticipated this conflict. According to the HCRA of 1989 and HCSA of 1993, future adjustments of payment should be better linked to costs and quality monitoring of outcomes. Concentration should also be on the quality of new medical technologies provided. Nevertheless, the problem remains: how should prices be adjusted to improve quality of health care while reducing overutilisation?

The years since the HCRA of 1989 have shown that price containment is difficult to obtain if there is inflation and lower economic growth. In this situation, the additional revenues are not available to pay the increased costs. Therefore, health care providers must use their abilities to induce demand and increase prices where possible.

The unification of the two Germanies has been considered and addressed by price-containment policy. Fee schedules for physician and dental services have been established in the five Eastern *Länder* of Germany, but with deduction of 45% of the conversion factor. Thus, at present, two different price levels exist. The two levels of fee schedules are being harmonized, step by step, along with the equalisation of the wage levels in both parts of Germany.

Despite of the lower fee level in the Eastern *Länder,* the majority of physicians have invested in private offices and are not staying in the former ambulatory health care centres. No wonder. The expected incomes from private practice are much higher than the former wages of physicians and dentists in the centres. It can be expected that the physicians in new offices and hospitals in the Eastern *Länder* will push utilisation to amortise their investments.

In future, one of the major problems of the German health care system will be to provide adequate services for patients in need of nursing care. The government has announced the establishment of a new social fund for nursing care from the beginning of 1993, to be financed equally by the employees and employers. Expenditures for long-term care in nursing homes, and for home care, are the fastest growing expenses in health care. In the nursing care area, comparable reimbursement regulations like those in the other fields of the health care system are not available. At the moment, the organisation of nursing service providers is also very poor. Nevertheless, Germany is already considering the application of the cost-containment experience to the field of nursing care.

Acknowledgments

The author is particularly grateful for the comments of Jean-Pierre Poullier (OECD), Leslie Greenwald, Peter Rosenberg, George J. Schieber, Mike Borowitz, G. Neumann and Alice Young.

Bibliography

In this article "Germany" or "German" refers only to the boundaries and population of the Federal Republic of Germany before reunification. Nevertheless, it should be noted that the characteristics of its health care system have been extended to the Eastern Länder from January 1, 1991.

BASYS and CREDES (1990), *ECO-SANTÉ*, Das Gesundheitswesen auf PC, Deutsche Version 2.1, Augsburg.

BASYS and CREDES (1992), *ECO-SANTÉ*, Das Gesundheitswesen auf PC, Deutsche Version 2.1.1, Augsburg.

Berg, H. (1986), *Bilanz der Kostendämpfungspolitik im Gesundheitswesen 1977-84*, Sankt Augustin, Asgard Verlag Hippe.

Beske, F. (1982), "Expenditures and attempts of cost-containment in the statutory health insurance system of the Federal Republic of Germany", in McLachlan, G. and Maynard, A. (eds.), *The public/private mix for health*, London, The Nuffield Provincial Hospital Trust, pp. 233-263.

Geissler, U. (1981), "Alternative methods of physician compensation and their effects on physician activity – an international comparision", *Country Report for the Federal Republic of Germany*, Paris, Centre de recherche pour l'étude et l'observation des conditions de vie (CREDOC).

Geißler, H. (1976), "Krankenversicherungsbudget '80'", Mainz, Ministerium für Soziales, Gesundheit und Sport.

Herder-Dorneich, Ph. (1980), *Gesundheitsökonomik – Systemsteuerung und Ordnungspolitik im Gesundheitswesen*, Stuttgart, Ferdinand Enke Verlag.

Kassenärztliche Bundesvereinigung (1990), *Grunddaten zur Kassenärztlichen Versorgung in der Bundesrepublik Deutschland*, Köln-Lövenich, Deutscher Ärzte-Verlag.

Kassenzahnärztliche Bundesvereinigung (eds.) (1990), *Statistische Basisdaten zur Kassenzahnärztlichen Versorgung*, Köln.

Neubauer, G. and Birkner, B. (1980), *Beeinflußt die Krankenversicherung das Verhalten von Arzt und Patient?*, in Sozialer Fortschritt, Heft 7/8, Bonn.

OCDE/CREDES (1991), *OECD Health Data*, Paris.

Rosenberg, P. (1986), "The Origin and the Development of Compulsory Health Insurance in Germany", in Ligth, D.W. and Schuller, A. (eds.), *Political Values and Health Care: The German Experience*, Cambridge, Mass., The MIT Press, pp. 105-126.

Schieber, G.J. and Poullier, J.-P. (1990), "Overview of international comparisons of health care expenditures", in *Health Care Systems in transition*, OECD, Paris.

Schneider, M., Sommer, J.H., Keçeci, A., Scholtes, L. and Welzel, A. (1990), *Gesundheitssysteme im internationalen Vergleich*, Ministry of Labour and Social Affairs, Research Report No. 160, 2nd ed., Bonn.

Schwabe, U. and Paffrath, D. (1990), *Arzneiverordnungs-Report '90*, Stuttgart-New York, Gustav Fischer Verlag, p. 9.

Sermeus, G. and Adriaenssens, G. (1989), *Drug prices and drug legislation in Europe – An analysis of the situation in the twelve Member States of the European Countries*, Brussels, BEUC/112/89, March.

Statistisches Bundesamt (1989), *Krankenhäuser 1988*, Fachserie 12 Gesundheitswesen, Reihe 6, p. 12, Stuttgart, Mainz, Kohlhammer.

PAYING FOR PRESCRIPTIONS IN EUROPE

by

Michael Dickson*

Introduction

Payment for prescription drugs is a part of health care coverage in all European countries. Experience with these policies, however, has not been presented in a format which invites comparison. Comparisons are especially timely, since many aspects of health care policy in Europe and elsewhere are under review or currently being changed. Also, with the virtual completion of a single market in 1993, the establishment of a baseline of policy experience is important. This chapter is an attempt to initiate a comparison of prescription drug pricing and reimbursement policies by providing programme descriptions and analysis in the form of a general model. Policies related to quality control and marketing approval are not covered since they are quite complex and have been covered elsewhere. A brief background is provided here as the basis for the report before reviewing policies as they were in 1990.

Pharmaceutical products have been subjected to government regulation since pharmacists first prepared remedies for sale, but the effort has intensified in the last thirty years. Regulatory intervention in the pharmaceutical market place appears motivated by the twin concerns of public health and economics. Public health responsibility includes insuring a safe and effective drug supply. It is also founded on the belief that availability of prescription drug products must be restricted because of the potential for harm and abuse if used without proper technical supervision. Economic controls inevitably follow when governments accept responsibility for organising and funding pharmaceutical services. Policies generally reflect an attempt to balance health care objectives with scarcity of resources. Protection of public health is also an economic issue: the inappropriate use of prescription drugs increases costs to governments through higher mortality and morbidity. Increased length of hospital stay due to drug misadventures is but one example.

Motivation for regulation

Health care expenditure has been more stable in recent years but still consumes a significant portion of national budgets, prompting governments to seek new answers to problems of balancing social priorities with available resources. Pharmaceuticals are only about 10% of expenditure on health care, which raises the question of why this category is given so much regulatory attention.[1] The answer reflects historical trends in the development of health care policy and current economic concerns:

a) *Costs are increasing:* Table 1 indicates that pharmaceutical expenditure has increased more rapidly than Gross Domestic Product (GDP) in most European countries since 1970. Also evident is the increased proportion of prescriptions paid by public programmes.

b) *Costs exceed the threshold for intervention:* a review of regulatory action suggests that expenditure approaching 10% of a budget will attract the attention of cost-conscious administrators.

c) *Use is often excessive and inappropriate:* there is a substantial body of literature to suggest problems with prescribing practices and consumption of prescription drugs. The prospect of reducing waste while improving the quality of care is an appealing possibility.

* The opinions expressed in this paper do not represent the views of the institution with which the author is associated. The author is indebted to Jean-Pierre Poullier who guided him through the institutional maze of European pharmaceutical policies and supplied part of the underlying quantitative background.

d) Control is relatively easy: prescriptions are seen as commodities rather than services. The former are generally easier to control than the latter.

e) Ideology: the pharmaceutical industry is large and very profitable. Profitability from disease has long been viewed as inappropriate regardless of the benefits that may be derived.

Table 1. **Pharmaceutical expenditure trends in the European community, 1970-1990**

(in percentage)

	1970	1975	1980	1985	1990	Mean
Share of total expenditure on pharmaceuticals in GDP (TRx/GDP)	1.0 9	1.1 10	1.1 12	1.1 12	1.2 12	1.1 55
Share of public expenditure on pharmaceuticals in GDP (PRx/GDP)	0.5 10	0.7 11	0.8 12	0.7 12	0.7 12	0.7 57
Share of total expenditure on pharmaceuticals in total expenditure on health (TRx/THC)	20.9 9	18.0 10	16.8 12	16.3 12	16.6 12	17.7 55
Share of public expenditure on pharmaceuticals in public expenditure on health (PRx/PHC)	14.8 10	13.2 11	12.0 12	12.5 12	13.2 12	13.1 57
Share of public expenditure in total expenditure on pharmaceuticals (PRx/TRx)	57.3 9	60.1 10	61.8 12	61.3 12	62.5 12	60.6 55

Notes: The upper line supplies the arithmetic average of the twelve countries for which data are available, the bottom line the number of countries on which the mean is calculated. All calculations are based on current price values expressed in national currencies.
Sources: OECD Health Data, 1993; OECD Health Systems: Facts and Trends, Paris, 1993.

Cost is the unifying theme in this list of diverse reasons for regulatory action. Biotechnology may soon deserve a place on the list due to its promising role in new drug development, albeit at very high costs. Regardless, it is understandable that policy-makers apply price and reimbursement controls with the expectation that they will reduce programme costs, while improving the quality of pharmaceutical services.

Purpose and procedure

There is an extensive published literature on pharmaceutical expenditure, yet a significant gap remains for policy-makers because much of this work is only tangentially related to policies. This chapter attempts to fill the gap by merging published literature with new data to create a model of pharmaceutical expenditure described in terms of prescription reimbursement and pricing policies. The model is based on principles distilled from qualitative descriptions and supplemented, where possible, with empirical data on consumption.

Scope of the study

Europe was chosen for study because of the relative abundance of information concerning its long history of innovation in health care policy. The chapter compares data for the 12 member States of the European Community in 1990 to that for five other countries.[2] Among the latter, the Nordic countries (Finland, Norway and Sweden) are incorporated because of their geographic and cultural proximity to

Europe and of their candidacy to the Community while Canada and the United States are interesting in terms of their large pharmaceutical markets and regulatory strategies.

The analysis of policies and consumption data is limited to out-patient prescription drugs, which represent the largest share of public drug expenditure and are often the most therapeutically significant. Quantitative and qualitative data were obtained from a questionnaire circulated to the 24 OECD countries, supplemented by other sources. Among these are two reports prepared by the European Bureau of Consumers Unions (BEUC) for the European Commission.[3, 4] Details on questionnaire data collection and analysis are found in the Appendix. Other data are taken from published sources and from research institute reports.[5, 6, 7] General health care statistics were extracted from the OECD health data file.[8] Policy descriptions reflect conditions at the beginning of 1990 although significant policy reforms initiated in selected countries since then are briefly reviewed. A broader context for the discussion is given by including data from 1970 through 1990.

Policy co-ordination

The purpose of examining policy is to assess whether their objectives are being met and, if not, to provide groundwork for change where needed. This must always be within the broader context of health care and social policy. Perhaps the best illustration of the need for co-ordination of policies is the influence of physician access (determined by health care policy) on pharmaceutical expenditure (a separate and subsidiary policy). Physicians determine drug demand through the prescriptions they write, but the physician effect must be taken as a given in the specification of pharmaceutical policy. Likewise, policy decisions within the drug benefit programme can influence needs in other health care sectors and social programmes. Nevertheless, it is common practice for health service programmes (e.g. drugs, physician services, hospitals, etc.) to be directed by different administrators with separate budgets. Despite the logic with which individual administrators may respond to budget constraints, the fragmentation of programmes inevitably produces mixed results.

Policy objectives

In addition to the need for programmes that will contribute to a common objective, the individual programmes must also meet their own specific objectives. Hurst[9] has listed five common objectives for health care policies: adequacy and equity in access to care, income protection, economic efficiency (macro and micro), freedom of choice for consumers, and appropriate autonomy for providers. In addition, a pharmaceutical benefit programme must be grounded in a set of objectives that are internally consistent while supportive of overall health care policy. Towards this end, the objectives of a drug benefit programme should be:

a) *Simplicity:* a drug benefit should be simple to use, to provide, and to administer.
b) *Accessibility:* a drug benefit must be affordable as well as geographically and therapeutically accessible. An affordable benefit is of little value if useful products cannot be obtained at reasonable locations.
c) *Budget transparency:* budgeting decisions must recognise the interrelationships between different modes of therapy and services. Health care and social services are inextricable.
d) *Innovation incentives:* the next generation of innovative pharmaceutical products depends upon an adequately funded research effort by research organisations and the pharmaceutical industry.[10] A drug benefit should provide compensation sufficient to support a fair share of the cost of innovation.

Clearly, policies governing pharmaceutical benefits should contribute to meeting these objectives. Reimbursement policies and objectives are targeted for analysis because these are the policies that bring together consumers, pharmacy providers, producers, and government. Pricing policies receive attention in the analysis because of their influence on consumption (demand), the need to set a price before marketing in many countries, and the issue of price transparency or harmonisation in the European Community market from 1993.

Procedure

The sections that follow give an overview of three topics before concluding with specification of a set of pharmaceutical expenditure models and conclusions based on them. First is a brief explanation of the components of pharmaceutical expenditure to illustrate policy options. Second is a review of the data on prescription reimbursement policies. These are the policies most visible to consumers. Finally, pharmaceutical pricing polices are reviewed. The discussion includes initial price determination for a drug, as well as derivation of the public price. A cross-country comparison on these two policy options is used to construct three policy models from which conclusions are derived and against which the previously specified objectives are measured.

The basics of pharmaceutical expenditure

In the current cost-conscious environment, perhaps the most difficult task facing prescription drug policy-makers is to set the limit on programme expenditure. Since expenditure is the product of an equation, expenditure = price x volume, conventional wisdom argues there are only two choices for exercising control. Implementations differ from country to country but the two universal policy options are price and reimbursement control. Typical components of these policies and their relationship to price and volume are shown in Table 2.

Table 2. **Policy instruments for controlling prescription prices and volumes**

Policy types	Main designed impact on	
	Price	Volume
Pricing controls		
Product prices	YES – direct	YES – indirect
Company profits	YES – direct	YES – indirect
Reimbursement controls		
Formularies	NO	YES – indirect
Cost-sharing	NO	YES – direct
Incentives for		
Prescribers	NO	YES – indirect
Pharmacists	NO	YES – indirect
Consumers	NO	YES – indirect

Source: Author's taxonomy based on conditions observed in 1990.

Pricing policies may set product prices at the time of marketing approval or control prices indirectly by setting profitability limits for manufacturers and importers. In addition to these direct effects, shown in Table 2, there is an indirect influence on volume through the traditional price effect on consumer demand (see Table 2). Direct and indirect controls are not mutually exclusive, indeed they are often found together.

Reimbursement policies are more varied and sometimes less direct. Limited drug lists (formularies) and consumer cost-sharing represent the major strategies for controlling volume. Incentives for consumers, prescribers, and pharmacists to limit drug use, are among the indirect modes shaping reimbursement policy. Because the latter methods are indirect their effect is difficult to assess and they must be regarded as supplemental approaches.

Pricing and reimbursement policies are clearly related. To predict their outcome, however, implies an understanding of the synergistic and possibly contradictory effects resulting from their interaction. The combined effects are not always predictable. For example, the over-the-counter (OTC) drug aspirin could be (in fact has been) removed from a list of reimbursed drugs in anticipation that consumers would purchase it themselves and thereby reduce programme expenditure. However, if prescribers change their analgesic prescribing behaviour (whether of their own volition or in response to consumer pressure to prescribe a reimbursed analgesic product), the likely result is that programme expenditure will increase (aspirin is a relatively inexpensive analgesic). The possibility for therapeutic misadventures increases, as more potent (*i.e.* prescription only) drugs are used. This in turn could further increase the cost of this policy change.

Conventional wisdom suggests that pharmaceutical expenditure can be constrained by controlling prices and volume. While the theoretical model is limited to these options, there are other possibilities (to be discussed later) which moderate expenditure growth by encouraging rational prescribing, dispensing and consumption. Macro-economic price and volume controls address only the economic component of drug use.

An overview of reimbursement policies

Table 3 reveals a limited number of reimbursement control mechanisms but considerable variety in the specifics of how they are applied. Nearly all countries have some consumer cost-sharing method. It

Table 3. **Pharmaceutical reimbursement policies for out-patient prescriptions, 1990**

	Payment when medicine is purchased	Consumer cost-sharing	Use of drug lists	Generic prescribing	Generic dispensing
Belgium	CON	CIN	CAT	NON	NON
Denmark	GOV/INS	CIN	PRD	NON	NEG
France	CON	CIN	PRD	NEG	NEG
Germany	INS	GPY *d*	PRD/CAT	POS	POS *d*
Greece	CON	CIN	PRD	NON	NEG
Ireland *a*	GOV	NCS	NX	NON	NON
Italy	GOV	CIN/CPY	PRD	NON	NEG
Luxembourg	GOV	CIN	NX	NON	NEG
Netherlands	GOV/INS	NCS	PRD	NON	POS
Portugal	GOV	CPY	NX	NEG	NEG
Spain	GOV	CIN	NX	NON	NON
United Kingdom	GOV	CPY *e*	PRD/CAT	POS	NON
Finland	CON	CIN	PRD/CAT	NEG	NEG
Norway	CON	CIN	CAT	NON	NEG
Sweden	CON	CIN	PRD/CAT	NON	NON
Canada *b*	GOV	NCS	PRD	NON	POS
United States *c*	GOV	NCS *f*	PRD/CAT	POS	POS

a) Refers to the GMS programme only.
b) Canadian programmes differing by province, refers to Ontario only.
c) U.S. programmes differing by state, refers to a "typical" Medicaid programme.
d) Applies only to products for where there is no "fixed price".
e) Though cost-sharing is an important principle for the NHS, in practice 80% of drug expenditure is for "exempt" prescription.
f) Medicaid allows states to use cost-sharing but this is not mandatory and it is used sparingly. See text for details.
Payment when medicine is purchased:
    CON = Consumer
    GOV = General government
    INS = Insurance
Consumer cost-sharing:
    CIN = Co-insurance
    CPY = Co-payment
    NCS = No cost-sharing
Drugs not covered:
    CAT = Therapeutic categories
    NX   = No exclusions
    PRD = Specific products
Generic Prescribing/Dispensing:
    NEG = Discouraged
    NON = Not encouraged or discouraged
    POS = Encouraged
Source: Author's estimates based on conditions observed in 1990.

is common for consumers to pay only the shared cost when receiving a prescription with providers receiving the balance from a third party, usually a governmental or quasi-governmental agency. Again, the mechanisms for this are varied. Formularies (or drug lists) are quite common but the size and composition vary widely. In contrast, there is little or no variability on the issue of generics: prescribing and dispensing are not encouraged. The theme of different applications of the same basic principle is repeated across the range of reimbursement policy options seen below.

Payment when the prescription is received

Providers are most often paid for their services directly by government or an insurance company. In three countries examined (Belgium, France and Greece), consumers pay for prescriptions and seek reimbursement from a government agency or insurance company thus creating a "liquidity trap". This "trap" probably has only a modest effect on prescription expenditure, but it remains to be fully documented. In theory, the liquidity trap represents a deterrent to consumption. In practice, however, it is more likely to affect expenditure. For example, the prescription purchase will be made, but because of the nuisance of filing a claim for reimbursement, the claim is sometimes not submitted. The appropriateness of this policy approach and the difference between intended and actual effect are interesting unanswered questions.

Consumer cost-sharing

Most European countries require consumer cost-sharing for prescriptions using either co-payment, co-insurance, or a combination. However, cost-sharing is tempered by the common practice of governments protecting some groups by methods such as limiting total annual cost-sharing, providing a complete exemption, or reducing the cost-sharing rate for selected groups or prescription products. Only the Netherlands has no consumer cost-sharing for prescriptions. However, a significant group of clients in France and the United Kingdom does not pay the cost-sharing mandated by their respective programmes. In France, this is mainly because cost-sharing for a large percentage of prescriptions is covered by non-public supplemental insurance carried by many people (in the early 1990s this was over four fifths of the population) and partly because certain beneficiaries are fully covered by the government plan (*i.e.*, their cost-sharing is zero). In the United Kingdom about 37% of the population are exempt from cost-sharing. This group includes, but is not limited to, pregnant women, children, the elderly, the unemployed, the poor, people with specified medical conditions, and people who have purchased a "season ticket". The exempt group is a minority of the population, but accounts for about 80% of prescription drug expenditure.[11] Thus, in these two countries at least, the intended effect of cost-sharing is diluted for a significant proportion of prescription expenditure. Consequently, France and the United Kingdom are classified, in the analysis that follows, as being without significant consumer cost-sharing.

Consumer cost-sharing is thought to have a salutary effect on expenditure in three ways: shifting expenditure from the third-party payer (*i.e.*, government) to consumers, reducing unnecessary drug utilisation, and increasing market efficiency by creating more cost-conscious consumers.[12] The second effect is problematic because consumers are not always the best judge of "unnecessary" drug utilisation. The third appears economically sound but, in practice, consumers have only limited ability to shop for drugs; especially the more expensive, single-source products. The first effect is straightforward but the exact outcome theoretically depends on the type of cost-sharing used. Co-payment (a fixed charge to the consumer for each prescription received regardless of the price) tends to impose a proportionally greater burden upon users of lower priced prescription drugs. The consequence is that average prescription quantity continues to rise in programmes using co-payment. Conversely, co-insurance (a set percentage of the prescription price) offers a disincentive to increasing prescription size, and creates some incentive for consumers to be wise buyers.

The use of cost-sharing on the one hand, and the upper limits to consumer spending for drugs on the other, demonstrate the limitation of this approach for containing pharmaceutical expenditure. It can be refined somewhat by targeting spending limits to high-risk groups or individuals with specific diseases. At some point, however, this begins to erode the principle of solidarity upon which many social programmes are based. Cost-sharing has a role to play but reason and experience suggest it cannot be expected to encourage rational prescribing, dispensing, or consumption which are the first principles of cost-effective use of pharmaceuticals.

Use of drug lists (formularies)

Only Portugal and Spain do not limit availability of either products or therapeutic categories of drugs. All other countries have specified either a positive or negative list as a means of controlling costs by precluding (or reducing, as in France) reimbursement for some drugs.[13] Although products excluded from coverage are not reimbursed by the health programme, they may be available in the market and can be obtained by paying the full prescription price. This does not mean paying the difference between a comparable reimbursed product and the excluded product, but means paying the entire prescription price of the excluded product. Formularies that significantly limit access to drugs are often controversial. Those opposed to formularies argue that patients are denied the full range of treatment options which in turn contributes to poor quality care. The removal of significant cost-effective care at one stage may ultimately contribute to increasing the overall cost of care, they argue. The opposing view is that reimbursing for every drug increases the cost of care and does not necessarily improve quality since only higher priced "me-too" and therapeutically ineffective products are excluded by a formulary.

Generic prescribing and dispensing

At the federal level, Germany has articulated a reimbursement policy encouraging physicians to prescribe generically. Government policy in the United Kingdom encourages generic prescribing but this is not incorporated into the reimbursement regulation. Nevertheless, the United Kingdom is cat-egorised as encouraging generic prescribing because a government system encourages cost-effective prescribing.[14] This effect has become more intensive as the new, indicative drug budgets have become operational in April 1991, which concern the largest family practitioner offices. In most other countries the issue is virtually ignored. France and Finland actively discourage generic prescribing through administrative impediments or reimbursement methods encouraging prescribers to write by brand name.

Policies encouraging generic dispensing are rare; only Germany, the Netherlands and Spain employ this practice. All other countries discourage generic dispensing either by not recognising the concept of generic equivalence or by specifying that pharmacists must dispense exactly what has been prescribed. The United Kingdom encourages generic dispensing to some extent by setting reimburse-ment limits for generically written prescriptions. If a prescription is written generically, it must be dispensed with a generic product for which a maximum price has been set. However, pharmacists are not allowed to substitute on prescriptions for multiple source products written by brand name.

In summary, 1990 reimbursement policies concentrate on formularies and, to a lesser extent, on consumer cost-sharing. Generic prescribing and dispensing incentives are rarely encountered. Formu-laries, by their nature, can be only marginally successful in controlling expenditure if the range of therapeutic categories (and products within categories) provides reasonable selection opportunities. It is therefore not surprising that reimbursement policies are coupled with pricing policies for controlling expenditure. Reference pricing approaches, adopted in the early 1990s, are making generics more attractive in several countries but the impact cannot yet be fully assessed.

An overview of pricing policies

All European countries included in this report exercise some form of price control over reimbursed products. Eight of the 12 regulate producer prices, and 11 countries set a limit to wholesaler or retailer margins (or both). Although *stricto sensu* price regulation is restricted to prescription medicines, in some cases it applies to non-reimbursed products and often a similar process exerts an impact on the price formation for non-reimbursed products. The systems of price setting tend to be complex with most countries developing prices based on some "internal" criteria; three countries have externally refer-enced pricing systems. Specific mechanisms are summarised in Table 4 and described below.

Type and scope of control

Only Denmark, Germany and the Netherlands allow manufacturers a free hand in setting product prices (in 1993, however, Germany mandated price cuts on products not on the reference price categories). New product prices in the United Kingdom are set by producers, but this capacity is

	Control description			Fixed margins	Wholesale margin %	Retail margin %	VAT rate %
	Type	Scope	Method				
Belgium	PCE	ALL	EXT	WS/RET	13.1 [d]	31.0	6.0
Denmark	None	n.a.	n.a.	WS/RET	7.8	29.8	22.0
France	PCE	ALL	INT	WS/RET	6.8 [d]	30.4 [d]	2.5 [g]
Germany	None	n.a.	n.a.	WS/RET	21.0	68.0 [d]	14.0
Greece	PCE	ALL	INT	WS/RET	8.0	32.5	6.0
Ireland [a]	PCE	OLD	EXT	WS/RET	15.0	C + F [e]	0.0
Italy	PCE	ALL	INT	WS/RET	8.0	25.0	9.0
Luxembourg	PCE	ALL	INT	WS/RET	15.0	33.4 [f]	6.0 [h]
Netherlands	None	n.a.	n.a.	* *	* *	* *	6.0
Portugal	PCE	ALL	EXT	WS/RET	12.5	20.0	0.0 [i]
Spain	PCE	ALL	INT	WS/RET	13.6	29.9	* *
United Kingdom	PRF	OLD	INT	WS/RET	12.5	22.0	0.0
Finland	PCE	ALL	EXT	WS/RET	* *	35.4	14.0
Norway	PCE	ALL	EXT	WS/RET	6.3	23.3	20.0
Sweden	PCE	ALL	INT	RET	3.0	27.0	0.0
Canada [b]	PCE	OLD	INT	RET	n.a.	C + F [e]	n.a.
United States [c]	None	n.a.	n.a.	None	n.a.	n.a.	n.a.

a) Refers to the GMS programme only.
b) Canadian programmes differ by province. Refers to Ontario only.
c) U.S. programmes differ by state. Refers to a "typical" Medicaid programme only.
d) Includes VAT.
e) Pharmacists add a dispensing fee to the actual cost.
f) However, a 20% discount to government-related plans is mandated.
g) Two rates apply: 2.5% for prescribed drugs, 5.5% for OTC.
h) Consumers also pay approximately 19% more in "contributions" to cover a variety of mandated charges.
i) VAT not charged on oral dosage forms.
* * Indicates missing data.
Type:
    PCE = Product price
    PRF = Company profit
Scope:
    ALL = All prices controlled
    OLD = Existing products only
Method:
    EXT = External reference
    INT = Internal reference
Fixed Margins:
    WS = Fixed for wholesalers
    RET = Fixed for retailers
Wholesale margin %. Retail margin %. Exact or maximum % allowed.
Source: Author's taxonomy based on conditions observed in 1990.

constrained by profit control guidelines that take the place of specific product price controls. Ireland does not control new product prices but differs from the United Kingdom in that specific prices for existing products, rather than company profits, are negotiated with producers. All other countries (Belgium, France, Greece, Italy, Luxembourg, Portugal and Spain) regulate prices of new and existing products. Procedures differ, but in each country the price must be requested and justified in writing.

Method of price determination

Belgium, Ireland and Portugal use an external reference system for setting product prices. The general principle is that prices within each country should not be significantly higher than other countries for the same or a similar product [after adjustments for import costs, currency and value added taxes (VAT) differences]. Also, more favourable pricing is sometimes allowed for products produced within the country setting the price. Among the countries using an external price reference system, only Portugal specifies the countries used for comparison (France, Italy and Spain or the country of origin).

The remaining six European Community member States (France, Greece, Italy, Luxembourg, Spain and the United Kingdom) use an internally defined pricing system. Some of these systems consider prices in other markets but the price calculation is clearly determined from internal considerations. Pricing systems generally start from a cost calculation, to which is added a "reasonable" margin of profit. This basic price can be adjusted for factors such as the value of exports, contribution to national employment, and research activity. The French method also considers the effect of the new product on the cost of health care, but the weight given to this factor is not clear. These pricing procedures, in general, conclude with a comparison of the government-calculated and producer-requested prices. When the price requested by the producer is rejected in favour of a government set price, the process provides for negotiation: legal appeals are always a possibility. Although internally and externally derived prices are both government controlled, there is a substantial difference in the philosophy which guides the process.

Applicability

In all cases observed, the price determination policy applies only to reimbursed products. There is, however, often a similar process for determining the prices of non-reimbursed products, or some linkage between the two markets. For example, price increases for non-reimbursed drugs in Belgium are governed by separate regulations. It is interesting to note that producers are permitted to set prices for non-reimbursed drugs, but the same is not true for reimbursed drugs.

Product types

Among the European Community member States controlling prices, only the United Kingdom does not set prices for generics. The British system also excludes the producers of branded products when their sales to the National Health Service are less than £500 000 per year. The hypothesis is that sufficient price competition exists among generic companies to keep prices reasonable and that there is a diminishing rate of return from price regulation.

Wholesale and retail profit margins

Controlled margins are expected in the regulated markets described above. Without controls on the final selling price of reimbursed drugs, the controls on producer prices would have little cost-containment effect. Since there is virtually no price competition on prescriptions, it is not surprising to find other regulations that set the location, ownership and numbers of pharmacies – with the intent of providing an adequate trading area to pharmacist retailers. Wholesale and retail margins are determined through negotiations between the relevant providers and government. This therefore makes them subject to the political process in which multiple priorities must be balanced by policy-makers.

VAT rate

Value added tax is charged on prescription drugs in all European countries except Ireland, Portugal and the United Kingdom. Where VAT is applied to prescriptions, the range was from 5.5% in France (it is now 2.1%) to 22.0% in Denmark. A discussion of VAT is included here only for completeness. VAT is not a major source of health programme funding, nor is it regarded as a deterrent to prescription purchasing.

The typical pricing policy relies on fixing prices from producer to consumer. Where this occurs, policy-makers have the necessary authority to strike a balance between pharmaceutical company profitability, and drug programme expenditure. Prices at the retail level are typically fixed throughout a country, and would be different only where there are differences in consumer cost-sharing. Thus, a comprehensive control on prices – combined with strong reimbursement controls – might be expected to provide adequate expenditure control. The models presented below demonstrate how reimbursement and pricing policies are used individually and in combination to form a comprehensive drug benefit plan. Comments on effectiveness of these policies for expenditure control are reserved for a later section.

Prescription payment models

Reimbursement policy model

The reimbursement methods described above tend to be found in a limited number of combinations which are described by three pharmaceutical reimbursement models: demand control, supply control and dual control. The demand control model relies primarily upon consumer cost-sharing and secondarily upon the "liquidity trap" in which consumers pay providers for prescriptions and then seek reimbursement. Of the two methods, cost-sharing is the more direct and effective. The supply control model uses limited drug lists and generic incentives (prescribing and dispensing) as control mechanisms. A limited drug list is the dominant form of control with generic incentives used infrequently. Combining the two primary control methods (consumer cost-sharing and formularies) yields a dual control model. Each model may be supplemented by secondary approaches. Salient features of the models are summarised in Table 5.

Table 5. **Pharmaceutical reimbursement model: taxonomy and classification**

Model traits	Types of models		
	Demand control	Supply control	Dual control
Demand side			
Consumer pays the provider	Possible	No	Possible
Consumer cost-sharing	Yes	No	Yes
Supply side			
Use of limited drug list (formulary)	No	Yes	Yes
Generic prescribing encouraged	No	Possible	Possible
Generic dispensing encouraged	No	Possible	Possible
European countries	Portugal Spain	France Ireland Netherlands United Kindom	Belgium Denmark Germany Italy
Comparison countries		Canada United States	Finland Norway Sweden

Notes: Countries are classified in the column corresponding to what is perceived as the predominant form of regulation. Ireland is mainly a "supply" control country but strict application of the guidelines shows that it also lacks certain supply controls.
Source: Author's classification based on conditions observed in 1990.

The country-level descriptions of Table 3 are used in combination with the above criteria to classify European countries according to the models of Table 5. Luxembourg, the Netherlands and Spain represent the demand control model where consumer cost-sharing is the only reimbursement method used to limit pharmaceutical expenditure. France, Ireland and the United Kingdom are representative of the supply control model because each has a formulary and none relies on cost-sharing to constrain drug expenditure (Table 3 indicates that France and the United Kingdom have cost-sharing provisions but, in practice, this affects only a small proportion of prescriptions). Belgium, Denmark, Germany, Greece, Italy and Portugal are examples of the dual control model. Within this group, only Germany encourages generic prescribing and dispensing as additional supply control measures.

Categorising countries according to the proposed taxonomy can be criticised as too simplistic. The intent, however, is to identify commonalties between policies based on dominant programme characteristics. It would be inappropriate to conclude that reimbursement policy is the only influence on drug expenditure, but it is reasonable to argue these policies are designed specifically for this purpose. A more complete picture of expenditure control is seen by including pricing policies in the discussion.

Price policy model

Price control methods tend to be more homogeneous than reimbursement controls. There is a simple dichotomy between policies that control producer prices and those that do not. Of the nine governments controlling producer prices, all but two (Ireland and the United Kingdom) control prices of new products and price increases for existing products. Table 4 distinguishes between controls based on external reference prices and internally derived prices. That distinction is not included in the following model, however. The model in Table 6 is based primarily on the single dimension of control type, since this is the most significant factor in price control while other descriptive factors exhibited little variability. A full control model applies to countries that control prices of new products and price increases for existing products. This is the most common approach in Belgium, France, Greece, Italy, Luxembourg, Portugal and Spain, for example. The next level of control is described as partial since only price increases of existing products are controlled. Ireland and the United Kingdom belong to in this category. Finally, there is a group of countries in which no control is exercised over prices for new or existing products. Denmark, Germany and the Netherlands are found here (Germany, as indicated, mandated price rebates in 1993).

Table 6. **Pharmaceutical pricing model taxonomy**

Full price control	Partial price control	No price control
Prices set for new and existing products	Prices set for existing products	All prices set by producers
Belgium	Ireland	Denmark
France	United Kingdom	Germany
Greece		Netherlands
Italy		
Luxembourg		
Portugal		
Spain		

Source: Author's classification based on conditions observed in 1990.

Composite model

Perhaps the best understanding of expenditure control can be obtained by combining reimbursement and pricing policies. Doing this provides the simple two-factor model described by Table 7. The columns of Table 7 describe the pricing policy model with three effect levels, table rows describe only the reimbursement policy, again with three levels of effect. Theoretically, those countries fitting the "dual reimbursement + full price control" description (lower left cell) will control pharmaceutical expenditure better than other combinations of policy options. Conversely, countries described by the "supply reimbursement + no price control" policy combinations (upper right cell) are expected to possess the least control over expenditure. Other levels in the model should be between these two extremes.

The data in Table 8 could, if circumstances were more favourable, be used to test the hypothesis implicit in Table 7. Problems with this are explained in the next paragraph after an explanation of the pharmaceutical expenditure data in Table 8. Table 8 shows pharmaceutical expenditure per capita in Purchasing Power Parity (PPP) adjusted US$. PPP-adjusted expenditure reflects the cost of purchasing a comparable basket of goods (in this case pharmaceuticals) in several countries, expressed in a common currency. Estimates of pharmaceutical expenditure in the national currency of each country were converted to US$ using the "Medical and Pharmaceutical Products" PPP index.[15, 16] PPP estimates of expenditure are preferred over those based on currency exchange rates because the latter are volatile and do not reflect inter-country differences in quantities purchased. Finally, to make inter-country comparisons possible the data in Table 8 are expressed as average expenditure per person using OECD population estimates.

Table 7. **Pharmaceutical pricing and reimbursement: composite model taxonomy**

Reimbursement controls	Pricing controls		
	Full control	Partial control	No control
Supply control	France	Ireland United Kingdom	Netherlands
Demand control	Luxembourg Portugal Spain		
Dual Control	Belgique Greece Italy		Germany Denmark

Source: Author's classification based on conditions observed in 1990.

The data in Table 8 cannot be used to test the proposed composite model shown in Table 7 because the latter has too many empty (and nearly empty) cells. A few observations about these tables will demonstrate the problems and suggest weaknesses in the model. If the cautions of the previous paragraph are ignored and the data from Table 8 incorporated into Table 7, it is apparent that the model is inconsistent with conventional wisdom. For example, average expenditure for countries with no price control is lower than for full control countries. Similar observations can be made about the reimbursement portion of the model. A more qualitative examination of Table 7 suggests that the differences may be less a function of sample size and more the product of culture, tradition, and economics.

A useful way to assess the poor predictability of the two-factor model is to identify those missing variables that would improve its performance if added. Among the more important variables to add are:

 a) exogenous health and economic policies,
 b) differences in effectiveness of pharmaceutical policies,
 c) differences in consumer preferences across countries, and
 d) differences in medical culture, especially prescribing tradition.

Table 8. **Pharmaceutical expenditure per capita at purchasing power parities, 1990**

(in US$)

	Total expenditure		Public expenditure	
	PPP	Rank	PPP	Rank
Belgium	303	6	185	6
Denmark	114	12	50	12
France	561	1	342	1
Germany	390	3	252	4
Greece	222	7	52	11
Ireland	162	8	110	8
Italy	440	2	292	3
Luxembourg	336	4	295	2
Netherlands	130	11	87	10
Portugal	152	9	106	9
Spain	332	5	204	5
United Kingdom	146	10	121	7
European Community	**274**		**175**	
Finland	189		90	
Norway	215		81	
Sweden	226		162	
Average Nordic countries	**210**		**111**	
Canada	269		72	
United States	210		24	

Notes: Pharmaceutical specific (not average) purchasing power parities are used. The area averages are arithmetic.
Sources: OECD Health Data, 1993; OECD Health Systems: Facts and Trends, Paris, 1993.

Each of these can account for some variation between the predicted and actual result obtained from the model. Although difficult to include in a quantitative model, the "missing" variables can be evaluated qualitatively by policy-makers. Viewed in this way, the model suggests the desirability of evaluating policies within the context of national cultural conditions (general and medical).

Overview of pharmaceutical expenditure

To this point, expenditure has been discussed only in an abstract way and with the implicit assumption that it was high and rising. This section reviews pharmaceutical expenditure of the 12 European Community States in three respects. First, a comparison of pharmaceutical price trends compared to other health goods; then an examination of pharmaceutical expenditure relative to other branches of the economy; and, lastly, an analysis of expenditure as a function of price and volume.

Pharmaceuticals and other health goods

In Table 9 the pharmaceutical price index is compared to indices of in-patient and ambulatory care for the period 1970-1990. It shows that all indices have increased. But the prescription drug index rose most sharply in the 1970s and stabilised during the 1980s. By this measure, pharmaceutical prices have increased less in recent years than have in-patient services and ambulatory care. Policy implications of this observed shift are not clear, since composition of the health care basket of goods and services has shifted over the years.

Caution should be exercised when making direct comparisons of prescription prices to those for other health care services: prescriptions are structurally very different from either ambulatory or in-patient care. A prescription, in every instance, is composed of an ingredient (a specific drug product) and a pharmacist's service. the producer share averages about 50% of the retail prescription price, with the balance covering other dispensing costs and the pharmacy's financial return. In contrast, ambulatory and in-patient care are predominantly services. Products may be used in the performance of these services, but they are incidental compared with the service component. Another important difference is found in the relative cost per unit of care. Prescriptions tend to have a low unit cost whereas ambulatory care, and especially in-patient care, have a relatively high unit cost. Shifts in prescription prices are potentially due to product or service costs, which are indistinguishable when total expenditure is the unit of analysis. More information is needed to make well-informed policy decisions.

Differences in unit price also complicate interpretation of results because, although prescription price changes may be small (per unit), the relatively high volume of prescriptions has a large multiplier

Table 9. **Expenditure index for pharmaceuticals, in-patient care and ambulatory care, 1970-1990**

(1985 = 100)

Indices	1970	1975	1980	1985	1990
Pharmaceuticals:					
Europe	36.7	45.6	62.8	100	116.0
Nordic	27.9	44.0	63.9	100	132.8
United States	40.3	46.3	65.5	100	142.0
In-Patient care:					
Europe	17.4	34.4	60.2	100	126.6
Nordic	24.9	43.2	65.1	100	130.0
United States	31.3	45.3	69.8	100	129.8
Ambulatory care:					
Europe	25.7	46.0	69.8	100	120.6
Nordic	26.3	34.9	59.4	100	138.6
United States	31.6	43.7	68.0	100	140.1

Sources: OECD Health Data, 1993; OECD Health Systems: Facts and Trends, Paris, 1993.

effect, thus considerable changes in expenditure. This is especially true where consumers are unaffected by the price increase, and there is no incentive to control consumption.

Pharmaceuticals and the economy

Three ratios of pharmaceutical consumption are offered to show nominal changes in pharmaceutical expenditure relative to general economic changes over time. At best, they indicate gross associations with policies and, at the least, they demonstrate the need for better data. Many government policies have changed over the years making it impossible to draw conclusions about earlier years based on 1990 data.

The ratio of public to total pharmaceutical expenditure (PRx/TRx) indicates how well a drug benefit programme protects clients against the financial risks associated with pharmaceutical consumption. If a programme is successful in meeting the pharmaceutical needs of clients, this ratio will be high, but in any case reflects rates set by policy-makers. Public expenditure on prescriptions as a proportion of GDP (PRx/GDP) attempts to capture the extent to which government policies have constrained growth in drug benefit expenditure relative to the general economic situation. Conventional wisdom suggests governments will desire to reduce this ratio while maintaining an acceptable benefit.[17] Finally, it is useful to know the ratio of public expenditure on pharmaceuticals to total public expenditure on health care (PRx/PHC) as a measure of a drug programme's position in health care delivery. This ratio can only be interpreted in the context of stated policies.

The anchor point for all comparisons in the report is 1970, since that year predates most health care system changes in Europe as well as the financial difficulties associated with the oil crisis that followed in 1973-1974. Since 1970, many changes occurred in health policies of individual European countries which cannot be disaggregated here to reveal specific associations. This period is also characterised by substantial changes in the service mix of health care programmes in Europe, changes which may affect total prescription expenditures relative to other economic measures. Two additional ratios – total prescription expenditure relative to GDP (TRx/GDP) and relative to total health care expenditure (TRx/THC) – help to put the three "performance" measures into a broader context.

TRx/GDP (refer to Table 1, line 1) shows there has been, on average, a general upward trend in pharmaceutical expenditure relative to the economy of each country. Line 2 of the same table demonstrates that public expenditure on pharmaceuticals relative to GDP, given by PRx/GDP, has increased substantially since 1970. This finding invites the question: What has the increased share of GDP purchased?

The next two lines of Table 1 show, respectively, that a decreasing proportion of health care expenditure, overall and in the public sector (TRx/THC and PRx/PHC) goes for prescription drugs. In combination with the previous ratios, it indicates that while pharmaceutical expenditure and other health care expenditure are on the rise, the latter is increasing more rapidly. The last line in Table 1 (PRx/TRx) shows a marked increase in coverage of the pharmaceutical bill for consumers through government-sponsored drug benefit programmes; much of this growth occurred in the late 1980s, following a modest decline during the 1970s and early 1980s. However, caution is required against arguing for a "sharp" upward trend. Again, the question is raised: What has the increased expenditure purchased? Is it due to higher prices or higher volume? Does the increase suggest new or improved therapies that reduce the cost of care in other segments of the health care market?

Change in pharmaceutical expenditure

The previous questions can be answered by separating expenditure into its price and volume components. At a macro level (aggregate volume by country), the results indicate sources of expenditure variation, without judging the relative value of expenditure for specific therapeutic categories.

A macro-level analysis of pharmaceutical expenditure was made for the period 1980-1990 using the OECD Health Data File and a well-known decomposition procedure.[18] To obtain the results in Table 10, changes in total pharmaceutical prices were removed from GDP price changes in each country (column 1). A similar method was used to adjust volume data to obtain the values in column 2. Finally, the volume changes were standardized for changes in population to reflect increases in real consumption per person (column 3). The same calculations were performed on public pharmaceutical expenditure with the results shown in columns 4 to 6. Column 6 (prescription drug volume per person)

Table 10. **Pharmaceutical expenditure growth in prices and volume, 1980-1990**

(compound annual growth rate)

	Changes in total pharmaceutical			Changes in public pharmaceuticals on expenditure			
	1 Price	2 Volume	3 Volume per capita	4 Price	5 Volume	6 Volume per capita	7 Volume per capita adjusted
Belgium	0.1	2.2	2.1	0.1	2.8	2.7	3.1
Denmark	1.2	0.1	0.1	1.2	−0.3	−0.0	−0.3
France	−3.4	8.2	7.7	−3.4	7.6	7.1	7.7
Germany	2.2	1.4	1.1	2.2	0.7	0.4	2.1
Greece	−4.3	4.4	4.0	−4.3	9.5	9.0	−0.5
Ireland	1.1	1.5	1.2	1.1	2.5	2.2	1.4
Italy	−3.9	11.7	11.4	−3.9	10.9	10.7	11.4
Luxembourg	1.1	3.2	2.8	1.1	3.3	4.4	3.2
Netherlands	−0.2	4.9	4.3	−0.2	4.9	4.3	5.4
Portugal	−0.2	2.1	2.1	−0.2	3.2	2.2	2.5
Spain	0.2	5.1	4.7	0.2	4.7	4.3	3.1
United Kingdom	−0.8	3.6	3.4	−0.8	6.4	4.7	4.9
Average **European Community**	**−0.6**	**4.0**	**3.7**	**−0.6**	**4.7**	**3.2**	**3.9**
Finland	1.4	2.5	2.1	1.4	2.7	2.3	2.9
Norway	0.9	1.7	1.7	0.9	1.0	0.6	−1.6
Sweden	−2.2	5.6	5.6	−2.2	5.9	5.6	5.6
Average **Nordic countries**	**0.0**	**3.3**	**3.1**	**0.0**	**6.2**	**2.8**	**2.3**
Canada	4.4	5.1	4.0	4.4	6.7	5.6	3.9
United States	3.8	0.5	0.5	3.8	5.4	4.4	2.4

Notes: The area averages are arithmetic.
  Columns 1 and 4: Excess (deficit) of pharmaceutical price growth over growth in GDP prices.
  Column 7: Pharmaceutical benefit per person net of coverage and cost-sharing in public programmes.
Sources: OECD Health Data, 1993; *OECD Health Systems: Facts and Trends,* Paris, 1993.

was further adjusted to reflect changes in programme coverage (*i.e.*, percentage of the population covered) and extent of consumer cost-sharing. The adjusted volume per person figure is shown in column 7 as the average consumption per person in publicly funded programmes.

The results, summarised in the European Community average, indicate that rising expenditure is the result of greater volume rather than price increases. Price levels fell 0.6% during the ten-year period while per person and total consumption increased. Total volume increased faster than per person volume, suggesting an expanding group of users rather than increased individual consumption. In the aggregate and from a limited perspective, the results imply that pricing policies have succeeded in controlling prices, while the effectiveness of reimbursement controls are open to question. However, the consumption increase should not be condemned without some assessment of the value received. If, for example, increased drug consumption represents a substitution for more expensive, less effective, or more hazardous procedures, this would be regarded as a positive development. Conversely, if the increase is due to unnecessary consumption that only increases total health care costs, the result should be deplored. Only anecdotal evidence exists to support either point of view.

Pharmaceutical consumption

Drug use review

An examination of appropriate drug use is beyond the scope of this report. However, questions raised in the previous section require some attention to broaden the current selection of policy options, and to address the matter of value received for rising drug expenditure. A cross-country comparison of drug use by therapeutic category is a useful analytical tool for answering such questions, since it associates consumption patterns with cultural and policy differences. An additional benefit of such an analytical strategy is that volume is seen in a therapeutically meaningful way rather than simply as one part of the expenditure equation. That is, the appropriateness of volume may be judged not solely by its influence on expenditure but in relationship to a therapeutically justifiable standard.

Unfortunately, data for such comparisons are not readily available in many countries. Thus, this section uses four countries for which data are available, to demonstrate the policy implications for therapeutic specific cross-country comparisons. Cross-country comparisons are difficult because of differences in drugs marketed and variations among the same products: dosage form, strength, and package size. The key to achieving a common unit of measurement is found in the Anatomic Therapeutic Classification (ATC) system combined with "daily defined dosage" (DDD) measurements.[19, 20] ATC classifications make it possible to capture all drug therapy for a given condition, while DDDs provide a standard unit of use. The DDD is interpreted as the number of "daily defined doses" per 1 000 adult population, and gives a rough estimate of the exposure of ambulatory population to an ATC drug class. To estimate the number of patients treated with agents in an ATC class requires information on duration of therapy.[21]

The ATC for cardiovascular drugs, composed of six sub-categories, is used for this illustration because it represents a significant therapeutic and economic grouping in virtually every country. Sub-category DDDs were obtained for five countries: Denmark, Finland, Iceland, Norway and Sweden. Table 11 presents a comparison of DDDs for four ATC cardiovascular categories. Differences across the categories are immediately obvious, but clear interpretations cannot be made since data are incomplete for the general cardiovascular category. Higher incidence of cardiovascular disease can account for some of the difference but variations in medical practice, cultural variations, and health care policies unrelated to pharmaceutical reimbursement are likely explanations. Policy and quality of care issues are brought into focus by such an analysis, and expenditure concerns can be given broader consideration. Why do differences exist? Are they economically and therapeutically significant? Are there implications for broader health care policy? Are policy changes needed to improve the quality of care?

Table 11. **Pharmaceutical consumption in the Nordic countries, 1990**

(defined daily dosage per 1 000 adult population – DDD)

Anatomic Therapeutic Classification categories	Denmark	Finland	Iceland	Norway	Sweden	Mean
CO1A Cardiac glycosides	9.5	24.1	6.1	10.5	16.7	13.4
CO1B Antiarrythmics, classes I and II	1.0	2.3	1.6	..	1.0	2.8
CO1C Cardiac Sympathomimetics and respiratory stimulants	1.6	0.6	0.3		1.1	1.1
CO1D Myocardial Therapy	7.4	24.9	13.8	16.2	19.4	16.3
CO1 CARDIAC THERAPY	**19.5**	**53.4**	**21.8**	**27.5**	**38.2**	**32.1**
CO2A Antiadrenergic agents (centrally acting)	0.6	1.6	0.3	2.4	0.2	1.0
CO2B Antiadrenergic agents (ganglion-blocking)	0.7	..		2.3	..	..
CO2C Antiadrenergic agents (peripherally acting)	1.2	3.9	0.7	5.4	0.8	2.4
CO2D Arteriolar smooth muscle (agents acting on)	12.2	20.1	13.2	15.9	20.2	16.3
CO2E Renin-angiotensin system (agents acting on)	4.3	12.3	10.3	8.0	7.8	8.5
CO2 ANTIHYPERTENSIVES	**18.6**	**39.1**	**24.5**	**31.7**	**28.8**	**28.5**

Note: The defined daily dosage is a statistical measure only and not a recommended posology.
Sources: OECD Health Data, 1993; *OECD Health Systems: Facts and Trends*, Paris, 1993. Nordic Council on Medicines.

Increasing quality and decreasing cost

The foregoing discussion suggests that price and reimbursement controls have been applied with some effectiveness but that the complexities of providing good pharmaceutical care cannot be adequately managed with these relatively rough controls. There is ample evidence to support the view that drug use is less than optimal and that total health expenditure could be favourably influenced by improving the way drugs are used. The work of Harris[22] in the United Kingdom and Avorn[23] in the United States represent two different approaches to improving drug prescribing. They are only a sample of the work done in this area. Both strategies begin with the premise that physicians will prescribe rationally when they have good information, and that rational prescribing is the most cost-effective means of containing drug expenditure. There is nothing inherently contradictory between this approach and controls placed on reimbursement and prices unless the latter are implemented in a way that inhibits the former. The confrontation is likely to be over budgeting, since physician information programmes have a cost and, given limited regulatory budgets, it is necessary to make choices.

A comparative analysis of Europe

At this juncture, it may be helpful to contrast European approaches to prescription drug coverage with selected countries elsewhere. Comparisons always provide insights and invite questions which will be all the more useful as a preface to discussion of European Community harmonisation and recent programme changes within Europe.

North America

The province of Ontario (Canada) and the United States follow the basic supply control model, with the addition of policies to encourage dispensing of generic drugs. In this respect, Ontario and the United States are similar to Germany, the Netherlands and the United Kingdom. The US Medicaid programme (see Tables 3 and 4) is described as not using cost-sharing, because it cannot be mandatory and those unable to pay are exempted. Only 20 states have cost-sharing provisions that range from $0.50 to $1.00 per prescription.[24] Although significant for some individuals, it represents less than 5% of the average prescription price, and many high-volume users are exempted.

The Canadian provinces of Manitoba and Saskatchewan should be mentioned since they have virtually universal coverage for prescription drugs. Unlike Ontario, however, they require consumer cost-sharing in the form of co-insurance. Both provinces also use a limited drug list and encourage generic dispensing by pharmacists. Their philosophy of coverage is more like that of Europe than Ontario's, but reimbursement policies show the North American propensity for use of generic incentives.

On pricing policies, there is more divergence between North America and Europe. Producers in Ontario are free to set prices, but competition exists in the form of government requests for bids every six months. This practice also fixes prices for a minimum of six months and protects retailers from the price squeeze experienced in the United States. Also, Ontario has compulsory licensing; this effectively creates a market even for those products under patent. A fixed margin is not established for retail prescriptions but reimbursement to pharmacies is limited to a dispensing fee, plus the cost of the lowest priced product in the therapeutic category prescribed. Saskatchewan is similar to Ontario in that it receives prices from producers which are fixed for six months and also places an upper limit (11%) on wholesale margins. Retailers receive a fee per prescription plus ingredient cost of the least costly item in the therapeutic category.[25]

The US Medicaid programme places no constraints on producer prices for new or existing drugs, nor are wholesale prices controlled. But Medicaid routinely places upper limits on reimbursement levels to retailers. Pharmacists complain that this practice places them in a severe squeeze between producer price increases on one side and the inability to pass on these increases on the other. Retailers are encouraged to use generic drugs when prescriptions are written generically and a Maximum Allowable Cost (MAC) programme encourages substitution of lower price products (usually generics) when the prescription is written for a multisource branded product.

An inspection of Table 12 shows large differences between North America and Europe.[26] The Medicaid programme is least like European countries. This is not surprising since Medicaid was designed to serve only the needy. In this respect, Medicaid is most like the Irish GMS programme in concept.[27] Consequently, the data for the United States do not approach the level of prescription coverage (PRx/TRx) provided in Europe. While some of the cost control methods are similar – and the reimbursement models have certain parallels – the basic difference in US health care policy is an equally important determinant of differences in drug programme policy and, consequently, in expenditure.

Table 12. **Summary of pharmaceutical expenditure statistics for Europe and North America, 1970-1990**
(in percentage)

		1970	1975	1980	1985	1990
Share of public expenditure	Europe	0.5	0.7	0.8	0.7	0.7
on pharmaceuticals in GDP (PRx/GDP)	Canada	0.0	0.1	0.2	0.2	0.3
	United States	0.0	0.1	0.1	0.1	0.1
Share of public expenditure	Europe	14.8	13.2	12.0	12.5	13.2
on pharmaceuticals in public expenditure	Canada	0.3	1.7	2.7	3.7	4.9
on health (PRx/PHC)	United States	1.7	1.8	1.6	1.7	2.1
Share of public expenditure in total	Europe	57.3	60.1	61.8	61.3	62.5
expenditure on pharmaceuticals	Canada	2.1	14.5	22.8	26.2	26.4
(PRx/TRx)	United States	5.5	7.7	7.7	8.3	11.1

Notes: Europe is an arithmetic average of the European Community countries with data (see Table 1). All calculations are based on current price values expressed in national currencies. "0.0" indicates a number less than 0.1%.
Sources: OECD Health Data, 1993; *OECD Health Systems: Facts and Trends*, Paris, 1993.

Nordic countries

The Nordic countries (while Denmark is included in Europe because of its European Community membership, it has a Nordic behaviour) fit the dual control model but do not have policies encouraging the use of generic drugs as do Germany and the Netherlands. The numerical comparisons of Table 13, unlike those of North America, are much more European in appearance. Public coverage of pharmaceutical expenditure (PRx/TRx) is lower to that in European Community countries while average coverage exceeds that of this area. Notably, the percentage of GDP expended for pharmaceuticals (PRx/GDP) in the Nordic countries is only about half that found in European Community countries; it has remained relatively constant, when compared to the European increase. Also, the proportion of public health expenditure devoted to pharmaceuticals (PRx/PHC) in the Nordic countries is less than half that of Europe. It has been suggested that this is because Nordic hospitals are larger than those in Europe, a fact which also may account for the relatively greater non-drug expenditure in the Nordic area.

Pricing policies in the Nordic countries are not unlike those in Europe. Every country controls prices of new products and price increases. An internal evaluation is used to set prices but there is an awareness of prices in other markets. Retailer margins are controlled so that the same product sells for the same price throughout a country. Sweden is one of the more interesting cases because retail distribution is government-dominated. However, the data and personal contact with Swedish authorities indicate that this arrangement has not totally insulated the system from rising pharmaceutical expenditure.

The Nordic comparison is interesting because, while very similar policies are in effect, these countries have been somewhat more successful in controlling expenditure. This may be cultural- or policy-related, but it raises interesting questions to pursue. Some of the answers may be evident in the next section, which examines some European policy changes since 1990.

Table 13. **Summary of pharmaceutical expenditure statistics for Europe and the Nordic countries, 1970-1990**

(in percentage)

		1970	1975	1980	1985	1990
Share of public expenditure on pharmaceuticals in GDP (PRx/GDP)	Europe	0.5	0.7	0.8	0.7	0.7
	Finland	0.2	0.4	0.3	0.3	0.3
	Norway	0.1	0.2	0.3	0.3	0.3
	Sweden	0.3	0.4	0.4	0.4	0.5
Share of public expenditure on pharmaceuticals in public expenditure on health (PRx/PHC)	Europe	14.8	13.2	12.0	12.5	13.6
	Finland	5.8	7.1	6.3	5.5	5.5
	Norway	3.1	3.4	4.3	4.6	4.1
	Sweden	4.8	5.9	5.0	5.5	7.4
Share of public expenditure in total expenditure on pharmaceuticals (PRx/TRx)	Europe	57.3	60.1	61.8	61.3	62.5
	Finland	33.7	46.5	46.7	44.5	47.4
	Norway	35.8	50.8	42.1	43.2	37.7
	Sweden	..	67.1	71.8	70.1	71.7

Notes: Europe is an arithmetic average of the European Community countries with data (see Table 1). All calculations are based on current price values expressed in national currencies.
Sources: OECD Health Data, 1993; *OECD Health Systems: Facts and Trends,* Paris, 1993.

Selected policy changes and proposed changes

Germany

In December 1988, the German Parliament adopted an act modifying (from July 1989) the prescription drug benefit, by introducing a "reference price" (*Festbetrag*) system for three categories of drugs, to be phased in over three years. Drugs in the first group are generically equivalent. The second group is composed of therapeutically equivalent products (especially where chemically related). The final group is a therapeutically-equivalent of combination products. This approach technically preserves the producer's right to set prices but discourages prices above the *Festbetrag* since consumer cost-sharing is required above the limit but not below it. To set a price above the limit is to risk losing market share. For the same reason, the system also encourages pharmacists to dispense products priced no higher than the reference price. Not surprisingly, the main point of disagreement between producers and purchasers (sickness funds) is where to fix the price. A high price renders no reduction in expenditure, and a low price drives producers from the market while potentially eroding the revenue base for research.

After six months of experience, nearly all producers of affected products (group one) had lowered prices to the reference prices, and sickness funds claimed significant savings.[28] Producers argue that the gains are temporary, that they are trivial compared to spending in other health care functions, and damaging to long-term viability of the industry. Nonetheless, the German government tabled another bill at the end of 1992 requiring some mandatory cuts in pharmaceutical prices. The conjunction of reforms implemented in 1993 lowered drastically that year's pharmaceutical bill.

The German experience since 1989 is an important policy landmark, and a model that others may emulate. To begin with, Germany represents a significant part of the European market; it also has a large pharmaceutical industry with a long history of unincumbered market prices. Note that the Netherlands offers a variation on the German model.

The Netherlands

On 1 July 1991, the Netherlands drug reimbursement programme was modified in a manner similar to that described for Germany with at least one important policy difference. Although the Dutch law also sets a "fixed price", it differs in that pharmacists are encouraged to dispense products lower than the upper limit because they are allowed to keep a portion of the differential between the actual and the reference price.[29] German pharmacists are, on the contrary, compensated by applying a mark-up on product cost, thus providing an incentive to dispense the highest-priced product under the reference price.

The Dutch method for fixing prices differs from that applied in Germany. In both countries, however, there is a concern that producers with very low prices would raise them to the limit, which could negate some of the expected savings. While the government has the power to set prices at a desired level, a concern for financial health of the industry places practical limits on the lower limits of reference prices.

The United Kingdom

From April 1991, a number of large family practices have been assigned Indicative Drug Budgets. While not a real financial limitation on drug expenditure for their prescriptions, prescribers exceeding their budget may be asked to explain why this was necessary. Peer pressure is provided through periodic reports mailed to prescribers detailing their positions with respect to other prescribers in the same region. While the scheme is too new to be evaluated, New Zealand's experience with a similar peer review procedure suggests that it exerts a strong short-run effect. A pilot programme of prescriber feedback prior to instituting the budgets suggested that doctors do modify their behaviour based on the comparative reports. Indicative Drug Budgets achieve their effect by encouraging prescribers to use generic or other lower-cost drugs to stay within budget. Consumers, by their demands for prescriptions, create another incentive for prescribers to use lower cost drugs. Physicians do not want to be constrained in treatment for financial reasons; thus, conforming to the budget insures two things: no administrative inquires that require time-consuming responses, and adequate pharmaceutical therapy for patients.

Spain

In December 1990, the Spanish *Cortes* passed legislation that will permit the executive branch to change at least three aspects of pharmaceutical policy, as part of a larger health care reform package. The first possibility is that of creating a negative formulary. Using this authority, policy-makers can exclude some drugs from reimbursement. Secondly, executive policy-makers may now choose to abandon the current price-setting system (which establishes prices for every product) and follow the British model, which sets profit targets. A third possibility is establishing reference prices as in the *Festbetrag* in Germany. Although none of these changes has yet been translated into regulations, they collectively represent an interesting policy strategy. Governments are becoming aware of one another's actions; they are more willing than ever to try new methods for controlling expenditure growth with less bureaucratic interference in the production and distribution of pharmaceuticals. Will policy-makers choose among the options or attempt to use all of them? What cultural adaptations will be necessary? Can policies be easily and successfully transferred from one country to another?

United States

In January 1991, a new "prudent purchasing" Act became effective in the Medicaid drug programme. It requires manufacturers to sign an agreement with Medicaid that obligates them to rebate to the programme a percentage of their Medicaid sales. By 1994, the "basic" rebate percentage will be 25% for brand name producers and 11% for generic companies. There is also provision for an "additional" rebate to cover pharmaceutical price increases that exceed the general inflation rate. Furthermore, producers are required to give their "best price" to Medicaid. In return for signing the agreement, Medicaid agrees that all products for a company will be reimbursed (11 categories of non-reimbursable drugs remain in effect). In the absence of an agreement, none of the company's products will be covered. The law appears to prohibit formularies, but implementation decisions have called this into question. Numerous implementation problems exist, but it remains an interesting policy experiment because Medicaid had directed all previous cost-containment measures at retailers rather than at producers. As in Germany and the Netherlands, there are concerns that companies will raise prices to compensate for lost revenue. Producers fear that reports of their Medicaid sales will not be accurate because they are to be determined from retail sales data.

An outcome of the debate was, however, a voluntary decision of several large manufactures to maintain the prices at which drugs are sold to purchasers acting on federal-mandated programmes.

France

In 1990, and in the early months of 1991, considerable discussion took place regarding the United Kingdom profit control system. A proposal has been made to adopt an *envelope* system, similar to the UK system, but with separate envelopes for "break-through" products. Meanwhile, short-term rebates have been demanded from the industry, the negative list has been enlarged, and a number of prices lowered.

Prescription benefit policies are changing in fundamental ways in several countries and the pace for change seems to be increasing. Policies from one country are readily transplanted to another in an attempt to find the correct regulatory mix. Market structures are being changed in an attempt to arrest rising pharmaceutical expenditure. The pending completion of the European Community market offers the likelihood of further change. The creation of medical references in 1993-1994 signals notably a larger reliance on effectiveness criteria.

This brief review includes only selected policy initiatives. Most countries have since 1990 modified one or more facets of their pharmaceutical regulations and reimbursement practices. The selection has been geared to address some of the most significant changes.

Harmonisation

Parallel imports

Since the beginning of 1993, the European market for pharmaceuticals is formally harmonised. This includes greater price transparency for pharmaceuticals and further parallel imports, the latter creating problems for research-based companies.[30] Parallel imports are now estimated at less than 5% of the market but companies fear this will increase as governments look for new methods of cost containment. The only course of action for companies to prevent parallel imports is to exclude the product from lower priced markets. For therapeutically important drugs, this may be regarded as failure of the company to meet its social obligations, and result in action to force marketing.

An alternative course of action (although not currently possible) would be to market a given drug at a single price throughout the European Community, and allow individual countries to adjust the price to consumers by whatever means they choose. Pharmaceutical firms clearly favour this course of action. Policy-makers, on the other hand, argue that this removes their most effective weapon against rising drug expenditure and virtually insures that expenditure will rise even faster. The possibility of countries setting a single price seems remote for historical, cultural and financial reasons. If policy-makers are content to allow, or even encourage, parallel imports, the absence of a common market will present serious problems.

Regulatory harmonisation

There has been some effort to achieve harmonisation of safety and effectiveness policies to improve the drug approval process. However, transparency in drug marketing policies seems distant for several reasons, including the belief that the Treaty of Rome does not require harmonisation in health care. If this pattern persists, there can be little movement towards a harmonised market for pharmaceuticals; national markets seem likely to maintain their current characteristics.

Meeting the objectives

Early in this chapter it was argued that a drug benefit programme should meet the tests of simplicity, accessibility and budget transparency, while creating incentives for pharmaceutical innovation. A few observations about adherence to these principles are suggested in the following review.

  a) Simplicity for consumers is often a question of how they will receive the benefit; by paying and filing a claim, or having the claims filed for them by the provider. It should be clear that any programme requiring consumers to pay for prescriptions and then file for reimbursement is more complex than one in which only net amounts are transacted with the provider (*i.e.*, cost-sharing). Consumer-pay systems, at least theoretically, offer some cost control but at the expense of simplicity.

b) The objective of financial accessibility must be balanced with demand controls, since price effects operate in this market and could lead to waste and over-utilisation when there is no out-of-pocket cost to the consumer. Cost-sharing thus attempts to control unnecessary demand, while permitting adequate access to the benefit. With the exception of the Netherlands cost-sharing is universal. However, in every instance, there were exceptions to protect individuals for whom drug expenditures could become excessive. Cost-sharing is seen as a necessity to control unwarranted demand, more than a mechanism of funding the benefit.

c) Therapeutic accessibility is more difficult to implement. In principle, programme beneficiaries should have access to those products necessary for cost-effective therapy, but most countries have decided that limits must be imposed on availability – either for quality of care or for economic reasons. Thus, it is not uncommon to find limited drug lists that exclude very expensive drugs in a therapeutic category or completely exclude certain categories.[31] Few would argue the reasonableness of excluding therapeutically marginal products but denying access solely on the basis of cost could deny care that will, ultimately, increase total health care expenditure. Policies that encourage the use of generically equivalent products assume they will yield comparable therapeutic results (usually based on the principle that quality is maintained by the approval and quality control processes). Opponents in this policy debate focus on two issues: whether generically equivalent products are therapeutically equivalent and at what level cost becomes too high. The former is a technical problem while the latter is political.

d) Co-insurance, the most common form of cost-sharing, is theoretically more egalitarian than a co-payment system. The latter tends to fall heaviest on those purchasing many lower priced prescriptions: namely the elderly or people with chronic diseases. In the presence of deductibles and expenditure limits (commonly practised), it is difficult to discern differential effects between co-insurance and co-payment. In the countries studied, co-insurance was the most frequently used technique and was combined with co-payment only in Italy. In virtually every country, there was a consumer expenditure limit. To be compatible with the objectives of simplicity and accessibility, cost-sharing schemes must be easily understood by consumers. They must also guarantee access to needed therapy.

e) Judgements on budget transparency are difficult. Briefly, the intent of this objective is to make explicit the interdependence between drug budgets and other social programmes. For example, psychotropic agents have made it possible to release thousands of individuals from expensive custodial care mental institutions. Unfortunately, many of these individuals do not have the social services necessary for them to function independently and the success of one programme becomes the liability of another. There are also medical analogies in which pharmaceutical break-through products have reduced medical treatment budgets. Unfortunately, these "savings" are not transferred into the pharmacy budget where gains would be enhanced. Segmentation of budgets into drugs, hospitals, etc. is administratively convenient but creates a discontinuity between programme manager goals... and overall policy.

f) The regulatory and pricing practices of countries reflect the size and sophistication of their domestic pharmaceutical industry. Countries with only a locally important pharmaceutical industry tend to have higher prices than countries without a large research-oriented pharmaceutical industry. Price disparity has been seen as differential support for innovative pharmaceutical research, a few countries subsidising R&D through higher prices. The converse position is that much of pharmaceutical research is devoted to developing marketing advantages rather than innovative products. The rising cost of innovation nonetheless dictates a policy of equitable distribution of the cost.

Policy observations

Convergence

The volume of literature on international comparisons is increasing. There appears to be a great interest among policy-makers to explore and apply methods used in other countries, even though cultural differences may require some modification in approach to local conditions. This trend, together with concern for quality and cost of health care, has created an environment in which change is the norm. The dominant theme in recent years can be described as policy convergence. Judging from policies in 1990, and the changes occurring since then, it is clear that policies in Europe and elsewhere are on a similar course. European countries are introducing more price competition into the market, while the US Medicaid programme, for example, is taking a stronger regulatory stance with pharmaceutical companies. In all countries, most policy effort is directed at producers rather than consumers or other elements in the distribution channel.

Controlling supply

Prescription drugs are included as a reimbursed expense in the health care benefit of every country studied, underlining their important role in medical care. It is clear that most countries regard some drugs as more important than others. Certain products, although approved for marketing, are not reimbursed by the health programme or are subject to lower reimbursement than other (by implication) more important drugs. The process of differentiating between products (to set level of reimbursement or place a product on a list) is likely to become more sophisticated as cost-benefit and quality-of-life assessment methods are more widely adopted. The continuing need to control expenditure may encourage greater consumer cost-sharing for "less important" products if they are to remain available. The alternative to this approach is removal of these products from any reimbursement (*i.e.*, assigning them a different formulary status). The reasons are many, but the guiding principle is an attempt to maximise value for pharmaceutical expenditure.

Use of generic products has not been encouraged in Europe to the same extent as in North America. There are signs this is changing as parallel imports become more evident in the market, and incentives for prescribing and dispensing generics continue to increase.

Controlling demand

Significantly increased consumer cost-sharing (across the board) seems unlikely if the principle of accessibility is to be maintained. Differential cost-sharing as described above is more in line with this principle, and could be used to reduce demand. The practical difficulty with this approach to decision-making is the separation of essential from non-essential products. It seems little will be gained by concentrating on this side of the equation.

Controlling prices

The *Festbetrag* recently introduced in Germany and a similar policy in the Netherlands will be closely followed to assess long-term results and implications. The German "fixed price" reform has resulted in substantial price reductions, but more time is needed to assess the effects on total pharmaceutical expenditure as well as industry innovation. There has been considerable interest among European countries in the United Kingdom profit control system, because it is a much simpler process than establishing individual product prices and the pharmaceutical industry in the United Kingdom is very innovative. For many countries, following the British system would represent a major policy change; it remains unclear whether such a change is currently possible. The absence of price uniformity across national boundaries has the potential to create further problems for drug availability and innovation.

Rational drug therapy

Too little is known about pharmaceutical consumption. The technology for reporting drug consumption exists but has seen only limited application. Elucidating consumption patterns would be useful to policy-makers interested in both the cost and the quality of care. In the first instance, quantity consumed is an important determinant of expenditure, especially in those markets that control price. Secondly, appropriate use of drugs influences the total cost of health care directly (through the pharmaceutical budget) and indirectly through morbidity and mortality associated with inappropriate prescribing and use. A related problem is the absence of an international effort to measure health outcomes associated with use of pharmaceuticals. Outcome studies have appeared but these stand as examples of what can be done, not as the result of policies. A better understanding of the link between use and outcome is crucial to implementation of the "wise buyer" concept – a policy-making theory more in evidence each year with each new policy initiative.

Policies to enhance rational drug therapy were not evident in any of the countries studied. Rational drug therapy (ensuring that patients receive the right drug in the right amount at the right time) requires an ongoing educational effort with patients, prescriber, and pharmacists. Two policies are needed to move in this direction. The first is a drug use review programme to monitor trends and provide appropriate information to health professionals and policy-makers in the service of patients. The second, and more difficult policy to institute would be directed at improving the quality of prescribing and dispensing through an ongoing effort to provide appropriate drug information. Studies are beginning to accumulate to suggest this will require a face-to-face contact with prescribers on a regular basis. Programmes of this type have real costs which must be justified by real savings through improved quality of care. It would be easy to dismiss this as a professional responsibility of physicians, but structural realities of the pharmaceutical market and practice environment argue for policy intervention (implementation may indeed involve professional organisations).

Unresolved issues

Many topics could be raised but two above all others deserve mention. First is the issue of differential prices. Problems encountered here have been discussed, but solutions are not foreseeable in the near future. Allowing the issue to remain undecided will only make it worse, and add to the second unresolved issue: funding for innovation. The large differences in prices also mean that the burden of research is not shared equally. Here, there are more fundamental questions about how to pay for research, as well as who should set the research agenda. Differences in reimbursement philosophies and levels make it more difficult to conceive single production and marketing strategies.[32] It is encouraging to note there is greater international exchange among policy-makers. This will hopefully contribute to more timely and better solutions.

Conclusion

Many sectors of the European Community are moving towards a single market but the movement is much slower for pharmaceuticals. Distinct national pharmaceutical markets continue to exist since January 1993. This is not surprising since health care is very personal and culturally defined. The price differentials noted above and the consequences of the differences will, therefore, remain a problem. In contrast to tendency for markets to be fragmented, is the almost universal increase in the consumption of pharmaceuticals in the European Community (checked in Germany and in Italy during 1993, following strong regulatory and pricing changes). Earlier it was noted that this appears to be the result of a broader use of drugs in the population rather than increasing individual average consumption. The reasons for this are many but the trend argues for programmes to encourage rational drug use. Gains from these efforts will be seen in reduced health care costs because detrimental effects from inappropriate drug use will be decreased and appropriate use will be optimised. Even though prices may continue to be different among them, member States can co-operate on policies to improve drug use.

Annex

Data collection methods

Sample

In October 1990 a questionnaire on out-patient prescription drug regulation and consumption was circulated to the 24 OECD countries. Responses were supplemented by "in-house" information to provide the database for the study. The report covers the European Community member States with only scant observations on Greece and Luxembourg for which too little information was obtained. Included are Belgium, Denmark, France, Germany (*Länder* of the former Federal Republic of Germany only), Ireland, Italy, the Netherlands, Portugal, Spain and the United Kingdom. The Nordic countries (Finland, Norway and Sweden) and North America (Canada and the United States) are included for comparisons. Descriptions of Canadian prescription drug policies focus on Ontario. However, the reported data are for all of Canada. For the United States, only the Medicaid programme is analysed. Since Medicaid programmes can be different in each state, the descriptions represent a typical programme. Tables 8, 9, 10 and 12 relate however to the entire country and all programmes.

Supplementary data

In addition to data collected by questionnaire (and that derived from published sources), the report makes use of a variety of the OECD health data files in *OECD Health Systems: Facts and Trends,* Paris, 1993.

Limitations

Any international comparison is difficult because of financial, cultural and demographic differences across countries. Currency exchange difficulties can be surmounted by the use of purchasing power parities or by measuring drug use in units of drug consumed. Cultural differences are, by nature, more problematical to quantify and are largely beyond the scope of this report. But in a plea for more standardised international data, it will be argued that controlling for all other sources of variation permits closer examination of cultural effects. The reader should also remember that this report is based on preliminary questionnaire information and judgements from written sources. Finally, there is the problem of missing data. Rather than estimating the missing pieces, they have been omitted, which causes some discontinuity across comparisons. This more conservative approach was preferred to imputing the missing data points, except in Table 10 where the few imputed statistics appear unlikely to distort the general picture.

Notes and references

1. Poullier, J.P. (1990), "Health care expenditure and other data", *Health Care Systems in Transition,* Paris, OECD. Also in *Health Care Financing Review,* Annual Supplement, December 1989.

2. The European Community includes: Belgium, Denmark, France, Germany, Greece, Ireland, Italy, Luxembourg, the Netherlands, Portugal, Spain, and the United Kingdom. Data for Germany are limited to the *Länder* of the original Federal Republic of Germany (*Länder* in the former Democratic Republic are not included). The countries wich have applied for Community membership are: Austria, Finland, Norway, Sweden.

3. Sermeus, G. and Andriaenssens, G. (1989), *Drug Prices and Drug Legislation in Europe – An Analysis of the Situation in the Twelve Member States of the European Communities,* Brussels, BEUC publication No. 112/89, March.

4. Andriaenssens, G. and Sermeus, G. (1987), *Drug Prices and Drug Reimbursement in Europe: A Comparative Analysis in Nine European Countries,* Brussels, BEUC publication number 18/87, October.

5. Silverberg, R.R. (1985), *Drug Reimbursement Systems and their Costs in Denmark, Finland, Norway and Sweden,* IHE Report 5, Lund.

6. Young, P. (1990), *European Pharmaceutical Policies,* London, ASI (Research).

7. Schneider, M. *et al.* (1991), *Health Care Baskets,* A Study for the Commission of the European Community, BASYS, Augsburg.

8. *Health Care Systems in Transition, op. cit.,* and *Financing and Delivering Health Care* (1987), Paris, OECD. The health data file is available on diskette *ECO-SANTÉ OCDE/OECD HEALTH DATA,* and also in *OECD Health Systems: Facts and Trends,* 1993.

9. Hurst, J. (1992), *The Reform of Health Care: A comparative Analysis of Seven OECD Countries,* Chapter 1, "Introduction and Main Issues", Paris, OECD.

10. Innovation through research is the basis for progress in many areas but pharmaceutical innovation raises policy issues that are fundamental and difficult to regulate. For this reason, pharmaceutical innovation is given close attention.

11. Based on estimates from the Economic Advisors Office of the Department of Health. The 80% figure includes net ingredient cost (NIC), plus pharmacist remuneration and applies to England only.

12. Hurley, J. and Johnson, N. (1991), *The Effects of Co-Payments in the Prescription Drug Market,* CHEPA Working Paper Series #91-1, McMaster University, Centre for Health Economics and Policy Analysis, Hamilton, Ontario, Canada, January, p. 7. This report includes a review of recent prescription drug cost-sharing research literature. Note that "co-payment" in the report is referred to in the current study as "cost-sharing" of which co-payment is one type (a fixed charge per prescription).

13. A "negative" list generally contains pharmaceutical products which, though authorized for sale, are not reimbursed to the beneficiary (or are reimbursed at lower than the prevailing cost-sharing rate). A "positive" list normally refers to those products eligible for full reimbursement. There are instances where this terminology has been applied to a dual approval procedure: one for safety and efficacy, and a second for reimbursement. This results in an enormous "positive" list as in France. The former concept of "drug lists" is thought to be more widely adopted and it is the interpretation used here.

14. Physicians receive a quarterly report comparing their prescribing patterns to that of other prescribers. The report emphasizes cost and quantity of prescription drugs with the intent of reducing the cost of pharmaceuticals provided to NHS outpatients. For an overview of the system see, Harris, C.M. (1991), "The Effects of Instituting a Prescribing Data Feedback Service on General Practitioners in England", Paper presented at the First Workshop on Strategies for European Pharmaceutical Industry and Patient Interests, Brussels, 31 January.

15. Ward, M. (1985), *Purchasing Power Parities and Real Expenditures,* Paris, OECD, pp. 11-12.

16. *Purchasing Power Parities and Real Expenditures, 1990* (1992), Paris, OECD, Table 9, p. 50.

17. To preserve comparability over the long run, these data must be adjusted to reflect changes in population composition (*i.e.,* age and sex).

18. For a health care example, see "Overview of international comparisons of health care expenditures", *Health Care Systems in Transition, op. cit.* Also see Schieber, G.J. and Poullier, J.P. (1989), *Health Care Financing Review,* Annual Supplement, December, pp. 1-7.

19. *Guidelines for ATC Classification* (1990), WHO Collaborating Centre for Drug Statistics Methodology, Oslo and Nordic Council on Medicines, Uppsala, February.

20. *ATC Index Including DDDs for Plain Substances* (1990), WHO Collaborating Centre for Drug Statistics Methodology, Oslo, April.

21. *Nordic Statistics on Medicines 1987-1989* (1990), Nordic Council on Medicines, Uppsala, pp. 9-19.

22. Harris, C. (1991), "The effects of instituting a prescribing data feedback service on general practitioners in England", paper presented at the First Workshop on the European Pharmaceutical Industry and Patient Interests, Brussels, January.

23. Avorn, J. (1991), "Improving the Quality and Cost-Effectiveness of Prescribing: Good Ways and Bad Ways", in *Proceedings of the International Symposium on Cost Containment and Pharmaceuticals: Issues for Future Research,* Talloires, France, July.

24. *Pharmaceutical Benefits Under State Medical Assistance Programs* (1990), National Pharmaceutical Council, September, Washington, DC, p. 98. A compilation of programme descriptions and drug use data on all state Medicaid programmes. Medicaid is the only federal programme that pays for out-patient prescription drugs.

25. Much of the information on drug programmes in Canadian provinces is taken from Anderson, L.J. (1990), *Provincial and Territorial Drug Reimbursement Programs: Descriptive Summary,* Health and Welfare Canada, Bureau of Pharmaceutical Surveillance, October.

26. The data for Canada are national while the policy description is for *Ontario* only. A review of Canadian provincial programmes shows that Ontario has a relatively liberal benefit, and aggressive cost-control methods.

27. *Report of the General Medical Services (Payments) Board,* for the year ended 31 December 1989, Dublin.

28. Meyer, H.J. (1991), "Fixed amounts for drug reimbursement: an example for Europe?", paper presented to the First Workshop on The European Pharmaceutical Industry and Patient Interests, Brussels, January.

29. DeVos, C.M. (1991), "Proposed changes to the Dutch prescription reimbursement program", paper presented to the WHO Drug Utilization Research Group, Verona, 15 June. The current legislation allows pharmacists to keep 20% of the differential. There are plans to increase this to 33%.

30. A parallel import that returns to its country of origin is sometimes called a reimport. In general, a parallel import moves between two different countries with different prices for the same product.

31. Some systems, such as that in Ontario, permit dispensing of any product on the limited drug list but reimburse the provider only for the least expensive product. The retailers incentive is clear and compelling.

32. Poullier, J.P. (1992), "Quels obstacles à l'harmonisation subsistent encore?", in *Europe Blanche XIV, L'Europe du médicament à la veille de 1993,* Paris, October.

PHARMACEUTICAL CONSUMPTION AND PRICING IN OECD COUNTRIES, 1987-1991

by

Helena Brus

Pharmaceutical expenditure accounts for between 8 to over 20% of total health expenditures in OECD countries.[1] In order to evaluate the role of pharmaceutical consumption in total health spending, a pilot survey of these countries was conducted in August 1989. This survey was designed to collect information disaggregating the data into price and physical consumption. Thirteen substantive replies to the questionnaire were received. (See the Annex for a brief summary.)

International comparisons of pharmaceutical consumption suffer from problems common to other areas of measurement of health care expenditure, including definition, distinction between private and public sector, comparability, and valuation. Pharmaceuticals, however, possess a singular advantage: an internationally accepted classification system. This provides a foundation for the collection of more comparable statistics on consumption.

The Anatomical Therapeutic Classification (ATC), as modified by the Nordic Council, groups pharmaceutical products into thirteen main categories according to the body system on which they act (the fourteenth is a residual category). These main groups are further broken down into subdivisions, of which the third and, sometimes, the fourth level represent therapeutic classes.

Even though the ATC system is available and in use in OECD countries, two respondents to the survey relied on an internal classification system, Japan and the United Kingdom. Some countries were able to supply information on public expenditure only (*e.g.* Australia – Pharmaceutical Benefit Scheme Expenditure). Others gave only sales information (Belgium, Japan).

Due to the diverse classification systems used in the replies, it has not been possible to compare drug consumption in detail in a large number of countries. The replies have nonetheless allowed for construction of a table analysing the distribution of pharmaceutical expenditure among the top ATC categories, such as the Alimentary tract (A), Cardiovasculars (C), Antibiotics (J), etc., and over time.[2]

Although fragmentary, the responses indicate diversity in the patterns of distribution of spending among the main therapeutic categories. Consequently, the information was supplemented by a variety of other publicly available sources for seventeen OECD countries. The results have been tabulated and analysed initially for 1987 (see Table 1*a*) and updated for 1991 (Table 1*b*). They reveal both unexpected similarities and differences.

The 1991 update suggests a trend towards convergence in the pattern of spending. This is explained by the change in Japan's structure of consumption between 1987 and 1991 (it was most dissimilar from the other countries in the sample but now resembles the remaining OECD Member states). However, considering only the distribution of consumption by therapeutic categories, another dissimilar country, Denmark, has not moved closer to the others during the same period. Overall results for the remaining countries are inconclusive.

An adjustment for price differences between the major ATC categories of drugs is a necessary second step to separate volume from price effects. This is theoretically possible using the methodology outlined by the OECD and other international agencies with respect to the development of purchasing power parities.[3] To achieve this goal, the expenditure classification is provided by ATC, and the relative prices should be developed starting with individual products, aggregated to the main ATC level.

Highly disaggregated measures of volume based on the concept of Defined Daily Dosage (DDD) already exist. They have been systematically collected in the OECD Health Data File (notably for the

Table 1a. **Distribution of pharmaceutical expenditure by ATC categories, 1987**

(percentage of total outlays)

	A	B	C	D	G	H	J	L	M	N	P	R	S	V
Australia	14.5	2.0	25.3	4.9	5.4	0.9	11.9	0.8	8.6	11.6	0.7	9.8	2.5	1.2
Austria	16.6	2.3	26.5	6.1	4.4	1.4	11.3	1.4	7.7	10.2	0.2	6.4	1.3	4.2
Belgium	17.0	1.2	21.1	4.5	5.1	1.5	11.8	1.4	6.8	17.4	0.1	9.8	1.5	0.9
Denmark	14.1	3.0	14.4	4.3	5.8	1.4	8.5	2.4	6.2	22.1	0.3	10.9	2.4	4.2
Finland	19.1	1.0	23.8	5.4	4.9	0.9	8.4	1.1	8.6	12.1	0.1	11.8	1.9	0.8
France	17.0	3.5	28.3	4.0	3.6	1.3	8.8	0.7	5.2	12.5	0.3	8.2	2.0	4.7
Germany	16.8	3.4	29.3	6.0	5.7	1.7	4.2	1.5	7.2	10.6	0.1	9.5	1.4	2.8
Italy	19.7	5.0	19.5	3.7	3.1	3.3	11.4	0.8	6.0	11.0	0.1	7.5	1.7	7.3
Japan	17.5	3.7	16.0	3.1	1.8	1.8	21.2	2.6	10.6	5.5	0.0	5.7	1.7	8.8
Netherlands	18.7	1.7	24.2	4.9	7.5	0.8	6.6	1.3	6.7	12.0	0.2	12.4	1.9	1.1
New Zealand	12.1	0.4	23.5	7.6	6.0	0.8	7.9	0.7	8.1	10.7	0.5	18.6	1.9	1.2
Portugal	20.8	2.2	18.0	4.3	4.2	1.4	13.4	0.2	9.1	14.8	0.7	7.5	1.6	1.9
Spain	16.4	3.8	15.3	4.8	2.8	2.3	12.0	1.1	6.3	10.9	0.2	11.7	1.9	10.6
Sweden	16.1	4.0	17.2	3.7	3.6	2.0	10.5	2.7	5.2	14.4	0.1	10.1	2.8	7.6
Switzerland	18.5	2.0	18.8	9.2	5.2	0.8	6.3	1.0	7.8	14.2	0.2	10.0	2.2	3.7
United Kingdom	17.0	1.3	22.6	5.1	3.8	0.9	9.5	1.2	12.3	11.2	0.4	11.7	2.0	1.1
United States	16.2	1.7	20.7	4.0	7.5	1.0	8.2	0.9	7.2	16.3	0.2	10.1	3.7	2.5
Average	16.9	2.5	21.4	5.0	4.7	1.4	10.1	1.3	7.6	12.8	0.3	10.1	2.0	3.8
Standard deviation	2.1	1.2	4.4	1.5	1.5	0.6	3.6	0.7	1.8	3.5	0.2	2.8	0.6	3.0

A = Alimentary tract and metabolism.
B = Blood and blood-forming organs.
C = Cardiovascular system.
D = Dermatologicals.
G = Genito-urinary system and sex hormones.
H = Systemic hormonal preparations excluding sex hormones.
J = General anti-infectives for systemic use.
L = Anti-neoplastics and immuno-modulating agents.
M = Musculo-skeletal system.
N = Central nervous system.
P = Antiparasitic products.
R = Respiratory system.
S = Sensory organs.
V = Other.
Sources: OECD Pilot Survey, August 1989; SNIP; Farmitalia; PMA; SCRIP (various issues).

Nordic countries). DDDs provide a convenient measure of the volume of pharmaceutical consumption as distinct from price. They are established first at the individual product level but can then be aggregated at the desired level in the ATC classification. The 1989 pilot survey revealed that a lot of detailed information is available about price and daily dosage of individual products. It confirmed that there were differences among countries in the choice of the preferred product and its most common daily dosage within the same therapeutic category. Most respondents indicated their current use of the concept of Defined Daily Dosage (DDD) was used in their country in some way.

The DDDs, however, differ among the countries. This is particularly visible in the Japanese case: the DDDs are lower on a milligramme basis when compared with the other OECD countries. Thus, the use of uniform DDDs (as those pioneered by the Nordic countries) is inappropriate for the area as a whole.

The survey indicated that a common system of categories, such as the ATC, should be adopted to have comparable reporting of expenditure on pharmaceuticals among OECD countries. Since the ATC classification is now well established among OECD countries, most (all) should be able to adapt their national statistical reporting to correspond with this common system.

Once the overall pattern of spending has been established, specific ATC categories can be disaggregated into therapeutic classes of drugs for further study. Given a knowledge of individual DDDs, the expenditure on a particular therapeutic class can be expressed in terms of DDD per capita and compared among countries. The average cost per DDD could also be computed. The pilot survey demonstrated that this information is routinely collected for all individual pharmaceutical products not only in the five Nordic countries and in Germany, but also in other countries.

Table 1*b*. **Distribution of pharmaceutical expenditure by ATC categories, 1991**

(percentage of total outlays)

	A	B	C	D	G	H	J	L	M	N	P	R	S	V
Australia	15.3	6.1	21.8	4.7	5.1	0.8	12.1	1.9	4.9	11.0	0.6	11.9	2.4	1.4
Austria	16.2	2.9	24.2	5.4	5.7	1.8	11.3	2.6	6.7	10.4	0.1	7.2	1.2	4.3
Belgium	17.1	3.3	20.6	3.9	4.8	2.3	12.1	2.3	5.8	14.9	0.2	10.0	1.5	1.3
Denmark	13.9	3.5	13.7	4.8	5.8	2.0	8.9	2.3	5.1	21.8	0.4	11.9	2.0	4.1
Finland	18.2	1.9	22.7	4.8	5.1	1.6	8.9	1.4	8.1	12.4	0.1	11.5	2.0	1.4
France	16.6	5.5	25.7	4.2	4.3	1.3	11.1	1.4	4.6	11.3	0.5	8.1	2.0	3.4
Germany	17.7	4.9	24.9	5.8	5.9	1.9	5.2	2.0	6.2	9.9	0.2	10.6	1.3	3.6
Italy	15.9	6.3	20.0	3.2	2.7	5.5	10.3	3.4	6.0	10.8	0.0	6.5	1.5	7.9
Japan	16.4	6.1	16.8	2.7	1.8	1.9	17.8	1.7	11.0	5.6	0.0	7.2	2.3	8.7
Luxembourg	12.8	1.1	23.3	6.2	5.8	1.0	7.7	0.9	6.2	10.3	0.4	21.0	1.8	1.5
Netherlands	21.7	3.7	20.3	5.3	6.8	1.1	5.9	1.9	5.1	11.2	0.2	13.7	1.8	1.3
New Zealand	12.8	1.1	23.3	6.2	5.8	1.0	7.7	0.9	6.2	10.3	0.4	21.0	1.8	1.5
Portugal	16.9	3.3	19.2	4.6	3.9	1.6	13.9	0.4	10.5	13.9	0.5	6.7	1.5	3.1
Spain	15.1	4.5	17.0	4.7	2.2	4.8	12.9	2.2	5.7	9.8	0.1	9.5	1.6	9.9
Sweden	15.5	6.4	15.4	3.3	3.6	3.9	10.4	2.7	4.2	13.3	0.12	11.6	2.4	7.2
Switzerland	18.0	2.8	17.9	9.0	5.8	1.1	7.2	1.2	7.1	12.9	0.2	10.8	2.3	3.6
United Kingdom	18.5	1.7	20.2	5.2	5.4	1.3	8.4	1.5	9.2	10.8	0.4	13.4	1.9	2.0
United States	15.5	4.2	19.5	3.9	7.2	1.1	9.9	1.3	6.2	14.9	0.2	10.6	2.8	2.7
Average	16.3	3.9	20.4	4.9	4.9	2.0	10.1	1.8	6.6	12.0	0.3	11.3	1.9	3.8
Standard deviation	2.1	1.7	3.2	1.4	1.5	1.3	3.0	0.7	1.9	3.2	0.2	4.0	0.4	2.7

A = Alimentary tract and metabolism.
B = Blood and blood-forming organs.
C = Cardiovascular system.
D = Dermatologicals.
G = Genito-urinary system and sex hormones.
H = Systemic hormonal preparations excluding sex hormones.
J = General anti-infectives for systemic use.
L = Anti-neoplastics and immuno-modulating agents.
M = Musculo-skeletal system.
N = Central nervous system.
P = Antiparasitic products.
R = Respiratory system.
S = Sensory organs.
V = Other.
Sources: OECD Pilot Survey, August 1989; SNIP; Farmitalia; PMA; SCRIP (various issues).

Tables 1*a* and 1*b* summarise the breakdown of pharmaceutical market by main ATC categories in 1987 and in 1991. These tables are based on the results of the survey as well as other sources of information, including pharmaceutical industry associations' publications and SCRIP. The tables establish an order of magnitude (in percentage terms) of distribution by main ATC categories and a ranking of countries within each group. As both tables illustrate the same basic points, the focus is placed on the most recent, 1991, data for seventeen OECD countries, including the United States. The absence of a few OECD countries, such as Iceland, Luxembourg, Norway, but also Canada and Ireland, is due to non-accessibility of the data at the time of writing.

In the context of Tables 1*a* and 1*b,* the term "expenditure" must be interpreted with caution because the information is based largely on sales of non-hospital pharmaceutical products. As a consequence, the figures do not represent total spending on pharmaceuticals. This is the case also in the OECD health data files.

In addition to showing spending profiles of the seventeen OECD countries, their average was also calculated. If we had a complete set of comparable OECD data, this would represent the average OECD drug spending profile – a convenient tool for inter-country comparisons.

On average, the largest expenditure categories in 1991 are for: cardiovascular drugs (C) with one-fifth of the total; alimentary tract and metabolism medications (A), 16%; nervous system drugs (N), 12%; antibiotics (J), 10%; and respiratory (R), 11%.

Based on standard deviations (given in the last row of Tables 1*a* and 1*b*), the largest ATC categories are also the ones with the widest range of variation. The respiratory drugs (R) show the greatest degree of variation, followed by cardiovascular drugs (C), antibiotics (J), and the drugs for the nervous system (N).

OECD Member states range widely in consumption of medical care including pharmaceuticals. The study of variations in the distribution of pharmaceutical expenditure provides yet another manifestation of these differences.

Just as other estimates of pharmaceutical consumption, the study of pharmaceutical expenditure distribution provides only a partial answer to the key question: how do we identify factors which not only influence consumption but also affect public policy?

Although some differences in the percentage distribution of pharmaceutical expenditure among the ATC categories and among countries are apparent, it is difficult to grasp their combined impact.

Consequently, a method is proposed which allows for more consistent analyses of the differences of this type.[4] The information gathered for Tables 1a and 1b can be further improved and the method proposed applied to better data in the future.

In Tables 1a and 1b, seventeen countries are listed and tabulated using the expenditure breakdown of the fourteen main ATC categories (A through V). Thus, each country is associated with a sequence of thirteen independent numbers corresponding to the percentage distribution among the main ATC categories, which is referred to as country-vector.[5] Degrees of similarity or dissimilarity between any two countries can be measured by comparing the corresponding country-vectors.

The simplest such measurement is an angle between the two vectors, as captured by the correlation coefficient. If the angle between the two country-vectors is close to zero (correlation coefficient close to one), the vectors are almost parallel and the countries are almost identical. As the angle increases, the correlation coefficient gets closer to zero, and the countries grow increasingly dissimilar.

The correlation coefficients between any pair of countries and the average are shown in Table 2a (1987) and Table 2b (1991).

The correlation coefficients shown in both Tables 2a and 2b indicate a high overall level of similarity between the countries except for Japan and Denmark, the most dissimilar pair in the sample.

Between 1987 and 1991, Japan moved substantially closer to the other countries, indicating a possibility of a convergence towards a common distribution of expenditure (it cannot be precluded that the quality of the estimates improved during the interval). At the same time, Denmark retained or even slightly increased its "distance".

The case of Japan

Based on Tables 2a and 2b, Japan is the most divergent country in the group. Consulting Table 1b (1991), Japan's expenditure for anti-infectives (J) as well as for anti-neoplastic and immunosuppressives (L), is double or triple that of other countries, while considerably lower for cardiovasculars (C) and nervous system drugs (N).

Figures in Tables 1a and 1b are based primarily on sales values. Each therapeutic category covers a relatively wide spectrum of drugs. To seek a meaningful explanation of the differences, it is necessary to disaggregate the data into volume and price. Nevertheless, the limited approach taken here helps to isolate particular areas for further analysis. Some conclusions may be drawn even from highly aggregated data.

Japan's profile differs considerably from that of other countries in the sample, prompting to question whether these differences will diminish or increase in the future and, eventually, follow the trends seen in distribution patterns in the rest of the developed world.

Based on data since 1987, Japan's distribution of pharmaceutical expenditure has undergone a visible convergence towards the average pattern.

The continued growth of cardiovasculars, especially anti-hypertensives and anti-arrythmics, is expected to continue. This trend is reinforced by the demographic and epidemiologic changes in Japan. Since the Second World War, Japan has experienced a dramatic increase in life expectancy: for males, from 50 years in 1947 to 76 in 1991; for females, from 54 in 1947 to 82. This now exceeds the levels observed in other developed countries. Continued gains in life expectancy are forecast for the next two decades. In the year 2000, the percentage of the old (those aged 65 and older) in the total population is expected to reach 20%. By the year 2010, it will have risen to 23%.

Table 2a. Distribution of Expenditure on Pharmaceuticals among main ATC Categories, 1987

Index of similarity: correlation coefficients

	Australia	Austria	Belgium	Denmark	Finland	France	Germany	Italy	Japan	Netherlands	New Zealand	Portugal	Spain	Sweden	Switzerland	United Kingdom	United States
Australia	1.000																
Austria	0.974	1.000															
Belgium	0.951	0.919	1.000														
Denmark	0.779	0.727	0.918	1.000													
Finland	0.970	0.950	0.957	0.814	1.000												
France	0.962	0.980	0.924	0.774	0.950	1.000											
Germany	0.941	0.953	0.878	0.717	0.910	0.971	1.000										
Italy	0.891	0.932	0.904	0.775	0.910	0.932	0.867	1.000									
Japan	0.741	0.781	0.704	0.510	0.694	1.400	0.586	0.839	1.000								
Netherlands	0.954	0.932	0.940	0.810	0.989	0.948	0.963	0.888	0.625	1.000							
New Zealand	0.914	0.846	0.864	0.744	0.925	0.858	0.887	0.752	0.547	0.928	1.000						
Portugal	0.910	0.902	0.962	0.856	0.932	0.881	0.820	0.940	0.811	0.895	0.773	1.000					
Spain	0.819	0.839	0.849	0.785	0.845	0.846	0.762	0.940	0.834	0.817	0.770	0.875	1.000				
Sweden	0.885	0.890	0.942	0.900	0.906	0.919	0.841	0.956	0.760	0.892	0.803	0.925	0.956	1.000			
Switzerland	0.901	0.901	0.938	0.866	0.961	0.905	0.908	0.893	0.628	0.951	0.870	0.922	0.851	0.910	1.000		
United Kingdom	0.969	0.939	0.936	0.784	0.984	0.921	0.923	0.885	0.733	0.956	0.920	0.925	0.834	0.877	0.931	1.000	
United States	0.944	0.909	0.979	0.915	0.963	0.932	0.910	0.886	0.630	0.965	0.881	0.930	0.830	0.931	0.951	0.935	1.000
Average	0.975	0.966	0.975	0.854	0.986	0.968	0.937	0.950	0.756	0.971	0.899	0.954	0.901	0.955	0.958	0.971	0.971

Sources: OECD Pilot Survey, August 1989; SNIP; Farmitalia; PMA; SCRIP (various issues).

115

Table 2b. **Distribution of Expenditure Among Main ATC Categories, 1991**

Indices of Similarity: correlation coefficients

	Australia	Austria	Belgium	Denmark	Finland	France	Germany	Italy	Japan	Netherlands	New Zealand	Portugal	Spain	Sweden	Switzerland	United Kingdom	United States
Australia	1.000																
Austria	0.950	1.000															
Belgium	0.968	0.951	1.000														
Denmark	0.792	0.739	0.879	1.000													
Finland	0.959	0.960	0.973	0.819	1.000												
France	0.972	0.984	0.955	0.752	0.953	1.000											
Germany	0.933	0.952	0.911	0.729	0.963	0.957	1.000										
Italy	0.886	0.938	0.907	0.728	0.889	0.944	0.897	1.000									
Japan	0.787	0.820	0.773	0.527	0.758	0.800	0.700	0.851	1.000								
Netherlands	0.923	0.892	0.923	0.795	0.961	0.899	0.953	0.831	0.667	1.000							
New Zealand	0.897	0.825	0.848	0.741	0.903	0.831	0.881	0.716	0.598	0.886	1.000						
Portugal	0.911	0.937	0.957	0.815	0.936	0.919	0.854	0.899	0.865	0.843	0.752	1.000					
Spain	0.866	0.894	0.878	0.732	0.855	0.889	0.828	0.951	0.901	0.798	0.747	0.884	1.000				
Sweden	0.907	0.863	0.929	0.880	0.889	0.891	0.854	0.920	0.782	0.881	0.802	0.873	0.938	1.000			
Switzerland	0.909	0.911	0.933	0.850	0.963	0.898	0.934	0.838	0.695	0.960	0.865	0.901	0.831	0.878	1.000		
United Kingdom	0.938	0.926	0.944	0.798	0.989	0.912	0.945	0.848	0.757	0.969	0.920	0.911	0.841	0.876	0.964	1.000	
United States	0.961	0.936	0.983	0.901	0.970	0.944	0.923	0.877	0.730	0.933	0.871	0.936	0.846	0.924	0.945	0.947	1.000
Average	0.975	0.970	0.983	0.842	0.987	0.971	0.955	0.931	0.809	0.948	0.886	0.950	0.914	0.941	0.958	0.971	0.979

Sources: OECD Pilot Survey, August 1989; SNIP; Farmitalia; PMA; SCRIP (various issues).

The mortality rate due to cerebrovascular and hypertensive diseases is expected to decline as the rate of treatment for these diseases is increasing. The treatment for the ischaemic heart disease (traditionally lower in Japan than in other OECD countries) is also thought to be on the increase.[6]

The growing share of sales of cardiovascular products in the total, when compared to antibiotics, is associated with the higher rate of new product introduction in the cardiovascular area. New innovative products are awarded higher prices under the Japanese pricing system, while the older products experience price erosion over time.

If lower underlying demand is causing a shift away from acute and towards more chronic-type therapies (more in line with the rest of the OECD area), then the Japanese reimbursement price system could reinforce the trend towards lower average prices for antibiotics as opposed to cardiovasculars.

Under the current price reimbursement system in Japan, high prices are granted to truly innovative products which remain exempt from price decreases for about two years. After this grace period, prices are regularly reduced, resulting in deep discounts offered by the manufacturers to the various medical institutions including the dispensing doctors who profit directly. The discounts are offered via the wholesalers.[7] Companies in Japan must introduce a steady flow of new products to maintain high price levels. If there is a greater demand for cardiovascular drugs rather than antibiotics, the greater proportion of novel heart drugs (or cancer or cholesterol reducing drugs) will boost not only the volume of cardiovascular drugs but also their prices. This would gradually depress the sales share of antibiotics.

The case of Denmark

Denmark is the other country which stands out as substantially different from the others. As shown in Table 1b, in 1991, Denmark spent relatively less on cardiovasculars (14%) than other OECD countries but substantially more on the central nervous system drugs (22%). In this respect, Denmark is quite dissimilar from the other Nordic countries (only Finland and Sweden are shown in Table 1b).

Based on the detailed statistics available from the Nordic Council on Medicines (by therapeutic category and both in value and DDD terms on a per capita basis), Denmark consumed more central nervous system (N) drugs both in absolute and relative value terms. Volume of consumption of these drugs is illustrated by the number of psychotropic DDD per 1 000 population in Denmark compared to the other Nordic countries.

Over time (between 1987 and 1990), the relative utilisation of psychotropic drugs in Denmark as compared to other Nordic countries diminished, suggesting some degree of convergence. Also shown is the utilisation of antidiabetic, antihistaminic, cardiac glycosides and anti-asthmatic drugs for the Nordic countries.

Indications for future research

The examples above illustrate some of the requirements for future comparative studies of the differences in pharmaceutical consumption among the OECD countries. First, there must be a consistent system of drug classification such as the ATC. Second, attention must be paid to the breakdown of information into the main ATC categories in order to identify major differences in expenditure allocation.

This cannot be done without an adjustment for the differences. Once this information is available, one cannot only study the changes in expenditure distribution over time but also target specific subcategories. This would strengthen on a thorough knowledge of the mechanisms inherent in different medical pricing and reimbursement systems.

Comparable figures on pharmaceutical expenditures would, over time, permit identification of spending patterns. Convergences should be expected, due to socio-economic factors affecting the demand and the increasing internationalisation of the supply side. For example, growing consolidation of the R&D-based multinational firms means that innovative drugs are developed for the international market. The increasing homogeneity of new drug markets is assisted by ever-increasing rates of dissemination of news concerning product breakthroughs. This may be expected to produce: increasingly closer dates of introduction, more uniform usage of drugs, and more convergence in the prevailing price levels.

Annex

Replies to the 1989 questionnaire

A questionnaire on pharmaceutical consumption and pricing was sent to the administrations of the OECD countries in August 1989. Australia, Austria, Belgium, Finland, Germany, Italy, Japan, Luxembourg, New Zealand, Norway, Sweden, Turkey and the United Kingdom provided substantive replies.

Among them, the ATC system of classification (with some modifications) was readily available and used in the case of Australia, Germany, Finland, Italy, Luxembourg, New Zealand, Norway, Sweden and Turkey.

Belgium and Japan relied on sales by manufacturers as the basis for their answers. Belgian data were grouped according to the ATC categories (the figures include exports). The Japanese data came from the Statistical Survey on Pharmaceutical Industry Production Trends, which showed production and used Standard Commodity Classification for Japan (not ATC). The United Kingdom had data organised according to the UK Prescription Cost Analysis (using Drug Master Index and its main codes and sub-codes).

Germany provided the most comprehensive data, including listing of volume (DDDs) and value of sales for each product organised according to the ATC system. In addition, cost per DDD was also computed for each product.

Valuation of expenditure varied from country to country. Some values were given at the pharmacy retail price (*e.g.* Norway) and some based on manufacturer selling price or some other price level in the distribution system.

Detailed information was available at the narrower therapeutic category levels, with DDDs provided for individual products. Based on the products listed in the answers to the questionnaire, DDDs for the same product differed between countries.

Notes and references

1. *OECD HEALTH DATA* (1993); *OECD Health Systems: Facts and Trends* (1993), Paris.

2. Norway and Luxembourg are not shown due to unavailability of data for both years analysed, at the time of writing.

3. *Purchasing Power Parities and Real Expenditures* (1992), EKS Results, Volume I 1990, OECD, Paris.

4. Method proposed by Dr. Tom Brus, School of Computing and Mathematical Sciences, Oxford Brookes University, Oxford, England, who also performed all statistical calculations and analyses.

5. The fourteenth category, V, is the residual and thus is not an independent variable.

6. Yano Report January 1991, International Pharma Consulting Ltd, Tokyo.

7. The current system is undergoing a change at the initiative of the Fair Trade Commission, which will reduce the range of allowable discounts, will slow down the process of price reduction, and limit profits on the sale of drugs. Drug bill in Japan is estimated for about 30% of the total.

ALSO AVAILABLE

Series OECD Social Policy Studies:

Health Care Systems in Transition: The Search for Efficiency,
No. 7 (1990)
(81 89 05 2) ISBN 92-64-23110-5
France: FF140   Other countries: FF180 US$30.00 DM55

New Orientations for Social Policy, No. 12 (1994)
(81 94 02 1) ISBN 92-64-14056-5
France: FF120   Other countries: FF155 US$26.00 DM46

Series OECD Health Policy Studies:

US Health Care at the Cross-Roads, No. 1 (1992)
(11 92 03 2) ISBN 92-64-23780-1
France: FF60   Other countries: FF80 US$9.00 DM25

The Reform of Health Care in Seven Countries: A Comparative
Analysis of Seven OECD Countries,
No. 2 (1992)
(81 92 02 2) ISBN 92-64-23791-7
France: FF180   Other countries: FF230 US$46.00 DM74

OECD Heath Systems: Facts and Trends 1960-1991,
No. 3 (1993)
(81 93 05 2) ISBN 92-64-23800-X
France: FF380   Other countries: FF475 US$89.00 DM150

MAIN SALES OUTLETS OF OECD PUBLICATIONS
PRINCIPAUX POINTS DE VENTE DES PUBLICATIONS DE L'OCDE

ARGENTINA – ARGENTINE
Carlos Hirsch S.R.L.
Galería Güemes, Florida 165, 4° Piso
1333 Buenos Aires   Tel. (1) 331.1787 y 331.2391
Telefax: (1) 331.1787

AUSTRALIA – AUSTRALIE
D.A. Information Services
648 Whitehorse Road, P.O.B 163
Mitcham, Victoria 3132   Tel. (03) 873.4411
Telefax: (03) 873.5679

AUSTRIA – AUTRICHE
Gerold & Co.
Graben 31
Wien I   Tel. (0222) 533.50.14

BELGIUM – BELGIQUE
Jean De Lannoy
Avenue du Roi 202
B-1060 Bruxelles   Tel. (02) 538.51.69/538.08.41
Telefax: (02) 538.08.41

CANADA
Renouf Publishing Company Ltd.
1294 Algoma Road
Ottawa, ON K1B 3W8   Tel. (613) 741.4333
Telefax: (613) 741.5439
Stores:
61 Sparks Street
Ottawa, ON K1P 5R1   Tel. (613) 238.8985
211 Yonge Street
Toronto, ON M5B 1M4   Tel. (416) 363.3171
Telefax: (416)363.59.63

Les Éditions La Liberté Inc.
3020 Chemin Sainte-Foy
Sainte-Foy, PQ G1X 3V6   Tel. (418) 658.3763
Telefax: (418) 658.3763

Federal Publications Inc.
165 University Avenue, Suite 701
Toronto, ON M5H 3B8   Tel. (416) 860.1611
Telefax: (416) 860.1608

Les Publications Fédérales
1185 Université
Montréal, QC H3B 3A7   Tel. (514) 954.1633
Telefax : (514) 954.1635

CHINA – CHINE
China National Publications Import
Export Corporation (CNPIEC)
16 Gongti E. Road, Chaoyang District
P.O. Box 88 or 50
Beijing 100704 PR   Tel. (01) 506.6688
Telefax: (01) 506.3101

DENMARK – DANEMARK
Munksgaard Book and Subscription Service
35, Nørre Søgade, P.O. Box 2148
DK-1016 København K   Tel. (33) 12.85.70
Telefax: (33) 12.93.87

FINLAND – FINLANDE
Akateeminen Kirjakauppa
Keskuskatu 1, P.O. Box 128
00100 Helsinki

Subscription Services/Agence d'abonnements :
P.O. Box 23
00371 Helsinki   Tel. (358 0) 12141
Telefax: (358 0) 121.4450

FRANCE
OECD/OCDE
Mail Orders/Commandes par correspondance:
2, rue André-Pascal
75775 Paris Cedex 16   Tel. (33-1) 45.24.82.00
Telefax: (33-1) 49.10.42.76
Telex: 640048 OCDE

OECD Bookshop/Librairie de l'OCDE :
33, rue Octave-Feuillet
75016 Paris   Tel. (33-1) 45.24.81.67
(33-1) 45.24.81.81

Documentation Française
29, quai Voltaire
75007 Paris   Tel. 40.15.70.00

Gibert Jeune (Droit-Économie)
6, place Saint-Michel
75006 Paris   Tel. 43.25.91.19

Librairie du Commerce International
10, avenue d'Iéna
75016 Paris   Tel. 40.73.34.60

Librairie Dunod
Université Paris-Dauphine
Place du Maréchal de Lattre de Tassigny
75016 Paris   Tel. (1) 44.05.40.13

Librairie Lavoisier
11, rue Lavoisier
75008 Paris   Tel. 42.65.39.95

Librairie L.G.D.J. - Montchrestien
20, rue Soufflot
75005 Paris   Tel. 46.33.89.85

Librairie des Sciences Politiques
30, rue Saint-Guillaume
75007 Paris   Tel. 45.48.36.02

P.U.F.
49, boulevard Saint-Michel
75005 Paris   Tel. 43.25.83.40

Librairie de l'Université
12a, rue Nazareth
13100 Aix-en-Provence   Tel. (16) 42.26.18.08

Documentation Française
165, rue Garibaldi
69003 Lyon   Tel. (16) 78.63.32.23

Librairie Decitre
29, place Bellecour
69002 Lyon   Tel. (16) 72.40.54.54

GERMANY – ALLEMAGNE
OECD Publications and Information Centre
August-Bebel-Allee 6
D-53175 Bonn   Tel. (0228) 959.120
Telefax: (0228) 959.12.17

GREECE – GRÈCE
Librairie Kauffmann
Mavrokordatou 9
106 78 Athens   Tel. (01) 32.55.321
Telefax: (01) 36.33.967

HONG-KONG
Swindon Book Co. Ltd.
13–15 Lock Road
Kowloon, Hong Kong   Tel. 366.80.31
Telefax: 739.49.75

HUNGARY – HONGRIE
Euro Info Service
Margitsziget, Európa Ház
1138 Budapest   Tel. (1) 111.62.16
Telefax : (1) 111.60.61

ICELAND – ISLANDE
Mál Mog Menning
Laugavegi 18, Pósthólf 392
121 Reykjavik   Tel. 162.35.23

INDIA – INDE
Oxford Book and Stationery Co.
Scindia House
New Delhi 110001   Tel.(11) 331.5896/5308
Telefax: (11) 332.5993
17 Park Street
Calcutta 700016   Tel. 240832

INDONESIA – INDONÉSIE
Pdii-Lipi
P.O. Box 269/JKSMG/88
Jakarta 12790   Tel. 583467
Telex: 62 875

ISRAEL
Praedicta
5 Shatner Street
P.O. Box 34030
Jerusalem 91430   Tel. (2) 52.84.90/1/2
Telefax: (2) 52.84.93

R.O.Y.
P.O. Box 13056
Tel Aviv 61130   Tél. (3) 49.61.08
Telefax (3) 544.60.39

ITALY – ITALIE
Libreria Commissionaria Sansoni
Via Duca di Calabria 1/1
50125 Firenze   Tel. (055) 64.54.15
Telefax: (055) 64.12.57

Via Bartolini 29
20155 Milano   Tel. (02) 36.50.83

Editrice e Libreria Herder
Piazza Montecitorio 120
00186 Roma   Tel. 679.46.28
Telefax: 678.47.51

Libreria Hoepli
Via Hoepli 5
20121 Milano   Tel. (02) 86.54.46
Telefax: (02) 805.28.86

Libreria Scientifica
Dott. Lucio de Biasio 'Aeiou'
Via Coronelli, 6
20146 Milano   Tel. (02) 48.95.45.52
Telefax: (02) 48.95.45.48

JAPAN – JAPON
OECD Publications and Information Centre
Landic Akasaka Building
2-3-4 Akasaka, Minato-ku
Tokyo 107   Tel. (81.3) 3586.2016
Telefax: (81.3) 3584.7929

KOREA – CORÉE
Kyobo Book Centre Co. Ltd.
P.O. Box 1658, Kwang Hwa Moon
Seoul   Tel. 730.78.91
Telefax: 735.00.30

MALAYSIA – MALAISIE
Co-operative Bookshop Ltd.
University of Malaya
P.O. Box 1127, Jalan Pantai Baru
59700 Kuala Lumpur
Malaysia   Tel. 756.5000/756.5425
Telefax: 757.3661

MEXICO – MEXIQUE
Revistas y Periodicos Internacionales S.A. de C.V.
Florencia 57 - 1004
Mexico, D.F. 06600   Tel. 207.81.00
Telefax : 208.39.79

NETHERLANDS – PAYS-BAS
SDU Uitgeverij Plantijnstraat
Externe Fondsen
Postbus 20014
2500 EA's-Gravenhage   Tel. (070) 37.89.880
Voor bestellingen: Telefax: (070) 34.75.778

**NEW ZEALAND
NOUVELLE-ZÉLANDE**
Legislation Services
P.O. Box 12418
Thorndon, Wellington   Tel. (04) 496.5652
Telefax: (04) 496.5698

OECD PUBLICATIONS, 2 rue André-Pascal, 75775 PARIS CEDEX 16
PRINTED IN FRANCE
(81 94 01 1) ISBN 92-64-14213-4 - No. 46865 1994